DESIGN THINKING
Innovative Solutions for a Better World

Gunikhan Sonowal
Faculty of Computer Technolgy
Assam down town University
Guwahati, Assam, India

CRC Press
Taylor & Francis Group
Boca Raton London New York

CRC Press is an imprint of the
Taylor & Francis Group, an **informa** business
A SCIENCE PUBLISHERS BOOK

First edition published 2025
by CRC Press
2385 NW Executive Center Drive, Suite 320, Boca Raton FL 33431

and by CRC Press
4 Park Square, Milton Park, Abingdon, Oxon, OX14 4RN

CRC Press is an imprint of Taylor & Francis Group, LLC

Library of Congress Cataloging-in-Publication Data (applied for)

ISBN: 978-1-032-82437-6 (hbk)
ISBN: 978-1-032-83561-7 (pbk)
ISBN: 978-1-003-50995-0 (ebk)

DOI: 10.1201/9781003509950

Typeset in Times New Roman
by Prime Publishing Services

To
my Parents, Wife
and my Sisters.

Preface

Design-thinking is a human-centered method of problem-solving that places strong emphasis on cooperation, empathy, and creativity. It is a way of thinking and a method that can be used to tackle many different problems, from creating new goods and services to enhancing existing ones. Fundamentally, design-thinking is about understanding human needs and motivations, coming up with creative ideas, and iteratively testing and improving solutions through feedback and prototyping cycles. Design-thinking is a mindset that anyone can adopt to approach complex problems with a fresh perspective. It is not just for designers. Design-thinking assists teams in developing solutions that are more pertinent, efficient, and interesting by placing user needs at the center of the design process.

Chapter 1 contains a brief discussion about design. It explains different definitions of design-thinking and outlines its history. Benefits of design thinking are considered in the following section. The goal of design-thinking is briefly discussed and the final section looks at design-thinking applications.

Chapter 2 discusses four rules of design thinking, including the human rule, the ambiguity rule, the redesign rule, and the tangibility rule. 1. The Human Rule: emphasizes the importance of prioritizing human needs, behaviors, and emotions throughout the design process. 2. The Ambiguity Rule: necessitates embracing ambiguity as an important aspect of design-thinking thereby reframing complex problems and exploring multiple perspectives to find innovative solutions. 3. The Redesign Rule: emphasizes the iterative nature of the design process. 4. The Tangibility Rule: emphasizes the importance of making ideas tangible and concrete through prototypes or visual representations.

Chapter 3 discusses the five typical phases of design thinking—

1. **Empathize:** entails understanding the needs and perspectives of users by conducting research, interviews, and observations to gain insight into their lives.

2. **Define:** combines information gathered during the empathize phase to identify key issues and challenges that must be addressed.
3. **Ideate:** generating a variety of creative solutions will be generated to the defined problem.
4. **Prototype:** ideas are transformed into tangible representations that can be tested and refined.
5. **Test:** prototypes are tested with real users to gather feedback and insights.

Chapter 4 discusses case studies and real-world examples of how businesses and individuals have successfully used design-thinking techniques to solve complex problems and drive innovation. These examples will demonstrate the practical applications of design-thinking principles across industries and contexts. By studying these real-world examples, one can gain a better understanding of how design-thinking can be applied in different contexts and find inspiration for design challenges.

Chapter 5 looks at how ideation, prototyping, and testing are supported by tools and technologies used in design-thinking. User testing platforms, collaboration platforms, prototyping tools, and brainstorming software can improve the design-thinking process. Teams can more efficiently generate ideas, visualize concepts, obtain user feedback, and iterate on designs with the aid of these tools. The chapter provides useful insights into how tools and technologies may be used to spur innovation and produce user-centered solutions in projects by comprehending contextualization functions in the design-thinking process.

Chapter 6 explores the difficulties and pitfalls that teams may encounter when applying design-thinking. Resistance to change, lack of support from stakeholders, lack of resources, and difficulty in transitioning from a traditional problem-solving mindset to a human-centered approach are some typical challenges. The chapter provides teams with useful advice and best practices for overcoming obstacles and avoiding mistakes when implementing design-thinking, thereby enabling them to be more prepared to lead successful initiatives and projects.

Chapter 7 examines how design-thinking and futures thinking can be combined to produce a more comprehensive approach to innovation. By integrating design-thinking's human-centered approach and futures thinking's forward-looking viewpoint, teams can create solutions that address present user needs and predict future trends. Throughout this chapter, the team will discover how to stimulate creativity, foresee change, and make a lasting impression by utilizing the advantages of design and futures thinking. By adopting a proactive mentality and incorporating future-oriented factors into the design procedure, groups can remain ahead of the curve and produce solutions that are pertinent in the present, resilient, and adaptable for the times ahead.

Acknowledgement

I would like to share this happy occasion with my family, who are the greatest source of strength. My wife, Mrs. Gitimoni Chutia Sonowal, my parents, Mr. Nandeswar Sonowal and Mrs. Nilima Sonowal, my sons Mr. Mritansh Sonowal and Mr. Miransh Sonowal and my sisters, Jimpa and Simpa have been invaluable during these years. It would have been difficult for me to complete this task without their constant encouragement, prayers, and understanding.

Contents

List of Figures

List of Tables

Chapter 1

Introduction to Design-Thinking

Innovation defined as a product, process, service, or business model with two crucial characteristics, uniqueness and beneficial is essential for an organization's success and growth. However, if no-one uses something new and innovative, it serves no purpose. Innovation may be upgraded through the application of design-thinking to generate useful, significant solutions. Design-thinking has long been hailed as the key to creativity and the antidote to complacency. Smart businesses are increasingly embracing "design-thinking" in their quest to identify new growth opportunities. Design-thinking is a problem solving approach that emphasizes empathy, creativity, and collaboration. It involves understanding the needs and perspectives of users, generating innovative ideas, prototyping and testing solutions, and iterating based on feedback. Design-thinking can be applied to a wide range of challenges, from product design to organizational change, and is used by companies, nonprofits, and governments around the world. The process is iterative and flexible, allowing designers to adapt to changing circumstances and refine their solutions over time. Design-thinking is often associated with user-centered design, which puts the needs, and experiences of users at the center of the design process.

This chapter discusses the following topics:

- What is Design?
- Design-Thinking and its History
- Advantages of Design-Thinking
- Design-Thinking Goals
- Applications of Design-Thinking

1.1 What is Design

Design is the process of developing human understanding to address a challenge. It is a reference to how things and people interact. Given this knowledge, the results of design change according to the diversity of human cultures and lifestyles. Design can refer to rigorous design processes like product design, engineering design, graphic design, fashion design, and others in varying situations. The word design has been used since ancient times.

The term "design" is derived from the Latin word "designare," according to online sources. It means that designare is the intention to create a plan. It is believed that the word "design" was thus first used to refer to a plan on paper. In 1884, during the 16th year of the Meiji period, the book "The 'Yijiang' Rules of Watermills" was published in Japan. The terms "yijiang" and "design" were translated either based on their original Chinese character meanings or interpreted literally. In the early 20th century, the word "design" became commonly used. Since then, the definition of the word has steadily altered over almost 100 years. The fact that "design" can imply different things to different individuals is another attribute of the word.

Finding a precise definition of design is challenging. However, according to Steve Jobs, "the majority of people erroneously believe that design is what it appears to be. People think it is this veneer—that the designers are handed this box and told, 'Make it look good!' That's not what people think design is. It is not just what it looks like and feels like. Design is how it works". Hence, a common error is for people to believe that design is only what it appears to be (Walker, R., 2003).

The term 'design' can be both a verb and a noun. It refers to the practice of designing as well as the result of that action—the artifacts generated by designing—which are called designs. It also refers to the field of design as a whole as well as the creative experts who work on the project; designers. According to University, L. (2021), designers are employed in many different sectors, such as:

- **Graphic Designers:** communicate ideas by using visual components like typography, color, and imagery. Graphic designers need more than just computers. Creating visually compelling and targeted messaging requires a highly iterative design approach that involves working with a variety of media and materials.
- **Information Designers:** view graphic elements like imagery, type, shape, color, texture, and space as tools to simplify, organize, and communicate information. Information designers study, synthesize, and translate data into intuitive information systems that evoke a response and action in the viewer.
- **Experiential Designers:** create displays and environments that communicate a message or feeling within a physical space,

- **Interaction Designers (IxD):** Interaction designers explore how words, visual design elements, physical objects, motion, sound, and space, can improve user interactions with products, environments, systems, and services. An interaction designer is someone as curious about technology and user interfaces as they are about people and purpose.
- **User Experience (UX) Designers:** focus on the experience a user has with products, services, or environments—both digital (think apps and websites) and physical. They improve lives by identifying problems consumers have and then envisioning ways to solve them.
- **User Interface (UI) Designers:** use the research results from the user experience designers and interaction designers to sketch out what an interface will look like. Based on studies of how people navigate through a site, app, or tool, user interface designers plan and develop ways to make the navigation experience better.
- **Web Designers:** create functional, easy-to-navigate, and visually attractive websites. They make the overall look of a website fit with their client's brand as well as resonate with a target audience. Web designers need basic coding skills to communicate with developers, however, their main focus is on the organization, structure, usability, and visual design of a website. Working mostly on a website's front end—the colors, fonts, and aspects that users interact with—web designers use tools such as HTML, Cascading Style Sheets (CSS), and JavaScript to bring their designs to life on screen. They also ensure that websites are responsive, meaning that they work seamlessly across all device sizes and are accessible to users with differing abilities or disabilities.
- **Game Designers:** develop the layout, code, storyline, environment, characters, and sounds of video games. They might also create other immersive experiences where a player or viewer is at the center of the action, such as augmented reality (AR), virtual reality (VR), 3D audio, or using an LED wall to create a cinematic experience in a life-sized environment.

These are just a few examples of the various specialized domains in which designers work, based on their abilities and interests. They may also work in fields such as architecture, engineering, and industrial design. Designers can be employed by companies, agencies, or work as freelancers. The skills and principles of design-thinking can be applied across all of these fields and can assist designers in creating more effective and user-friendly solutions.

1.2 Design-Thinking and its History

The word "design" has existed since the early ages, however, Design-thinking first became prominent between the 50s and 60s. Knowledge of the roots and beginnings of design-thinking is crucial to understanding it. Design-thinking is a strong approach to meeting current needs for technological, strategic, and societal innovation in the modern world.

According to Dam, R.F. and Siang, T.U. (2022), "it would be nearly impossible to enumerate all the significant influences that contributed to the current understanding of design theory, method, and practice". The methods and procedures behind invention have been extensively researched for decades by business analysts, engineers, scientists, and creative people. However, World War II has had a significant impact on strategic thinking, and has since given rise to new approaches in handling challenging issues. It is perhaps true that this significant global event radically altered how people approach management, production, and industrial design in the contemporary day.

The article *design-thinking: State of Things* (IdeaKeep, 2018), places the root of design-thinking in the 1950s, when creativity approaches were first developed. Industrial Design—A Practical Guide to Product Design and Development by Van Doren (1954), which covers design methodologies and practices, was released in 1940. John E. Arnold first taught creative thinking at MIT in 1951 before moving on to Stanford in 1957. John E. Arnold was the first author to discuss the idea of design-thinking in Creative Engineering.

In the 1960s, Bruce Archer wrote several articles for the magazine *Articles in Design* that reflected his views on the various aspects of design and the necessity of approaching them methodically. The third editor of *Design* at the time was John E. Blake (L. B. Archer, 1968).

In 1961, a notable book, *Synectics: The Development of Creative Capacity*, was published by Gordon (1961). Generally, synectics is a strategy for solving problems that prompts ideas that the subject might not be aware of. Synectics, which is employed in design-thinking, utilizes the strengths of both the right brain (the dreamer) and the left brain (the reasoner), and it requires team members to be at ease navigating complexity and seeming contradiction.

Asimow (1962)'s *Introduction to Design* is considered a foundational work in the field of engineering design. Morris Asimow was the first author to consider morphology in engineering design. His approach was intimately related to the engineering philosophy he developed. He argued that design morphology proceeds from the abstract to the concrete not intelligible to the reader.

The book *Applied Imagination: Principles and Procedures of Creative Thinking* was written by Osborn (1963). He described the process of brainstorming in this book. The brainstorming process is crucial for determining what customers desire. Since customers need a variety of solutions to their issues, it can be challenging for them to determine which approach will best address those issues.

Jones & Thornley (1963) conducted conference on Design Methods. Alexander (1964) address the process by which a form is adjusted to the context of human requirements and demands in the first section of the book. In the second section, they offer a technique that enables the designer to use all of his creative imagination while avoiding the pitfalls of irrelevant preconceptions.

L. Archer (1965) presented his concepts at conferences for the design industry and wrote a book titled *Systematic Methods for Designers*, which was later published by the Council for Industrial Design in 1965 following a series in *Design magazine*. The method consists of six fundamental steps: programming, data collection, analysis, synthesis, development, and communication.

Simon (1969), a cognitive scientist and Nobel Prize winner, was the first to refer to design-thinking as a "way of thinking" and as a methodology. This was documented in his book *The Sciences of the Artificial*, published in 1969. Throughout the 1970s, he proceeded to make numerous contributions that are today recognized as design-thinking principles.

By the 1970s, design-thinking was able to gradually advance over the years by combining human resources with the technological and strategic needs of the time. It is currently regarded as one of the most cutting-edge methods in use.

In his 1972 book *Experiences in Visual Thinking*, McKim (1972), Emeritus Professor of Mechanical Engineering, also referred to the idea of design-thinking. In contrast to Simon, McKim is best defined as an artist and an engineer; "he concentrated his efforts more on the influence that visual thinking has on their capacity for comprehension and problem solving" (Dam, R.F. and Siang, T.U. (2022)).

Drawing on design research, Cross (1982) published a journal paper titled *Designerly Ways of Knowing* in 1982. In the paper, he contrasts the cultures of science, the arts, and the humanities with design cultures and demonstrates how design has its own intellectual and practical culture. This clarifies the statement, "There are things to know, ways to know them, and ways to find out about them that are specific to the design area." The paper establishes design as a field, the current conception in design theory, education, and practice.

In his book *design-thinking*, which Rowe (1991) gives a comprehensive overview of the process of designing in architecture and urban planning. He considers numerous, divergent theoretical viewpoints—whether they mandate forms or merely offer techniques for solving issues—as specific representations of an underlying framework of inquiry design.

In 1991, three industrial design firms are combined to create IDEO Design Consultancy. They were one of the first design companies to demonstrate their design methodology, based on design-thinking. David Kelley and his design company IDEO are credited with popularising the term "design-thinking". Design-thinking was approached by IDEO with an emphasis on empathy, collaboration, and prototyping. Companies throughout the world began to recognize and use this strategy.

Buchanan (1992) published the book *Wicked Problems in design-thinking* in 1992. In his book, he linked design-thinking and wicked problems. When handling challenges that are vague or undefined, design-thinking's iterative method is tremendously helpful since it reframes the issue in a human-centric manner, generates numerous ideas during brainstorming sessions, and takes a practical approach through prototyping and testing.

A paper titled *Task-centered user interface design* was published by Lewis & Rieman (1993). Task-centered approach is a subset of user-centered design, a method that enables designers to create and assess user interfaces in light of users' actual tasks. Lawson (2006) mentioned in his book *How Designers Think: The Design Process Demystified* that design is a process that can be supported with computers and by working in groups.

In 2004, Council, D. (2004) introduced the Double Diamond design-thinking process. It provides a framework for businesses to use design characteristics to find creative solutions and innovative ideas. It is divided into four stages: discover, define, develop, and deliver. Apple, Microsoft, Starbucks, and other companies have all used the Double Diamond design process. In 2019, an updated version of the Double Diamond was introduced that is agile and visualizes how it can fit within the organization (Elmansy, R., 2021).

The Hasso Plattner Institute of Design at Stanford (the d.school) developed the five-stage design-thinking approach, which is a non-linear, iterative process. The d.school lists these as the five stages of design-thinking: Empathize, Define, Ideate, Prototype, and Test, as shown in Figure 1.1. These five stages are still used today. This book primarily considers these five stages.

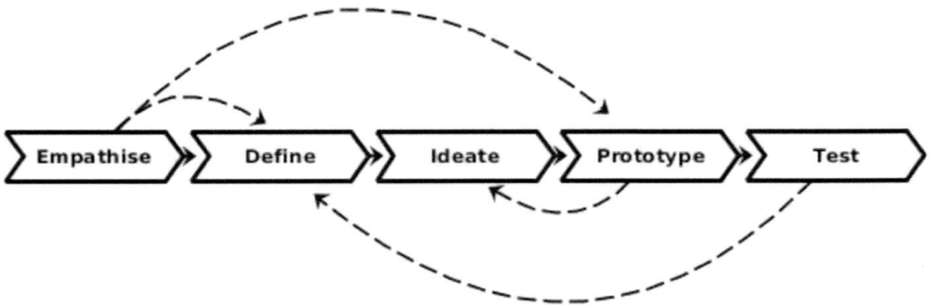

Figure 1.1: Five Stages of Design-Thinking

Over the last decade, the term *design-thinking* has gained a lot of traction in a variety of organizations and circumstances other than traditional settings. According to Renard (2014), design-thinking has roots in many different fields, and it is typically, but not always, connected to engineering, architecture, and related fields, in early design-thinking literature. Design-thinking is perhaps best characterized as a procedure and a state of mind put into practice to bring about constructive change in the world.

The basic concept is that the ways professional designers problem-solve are valuable to businesses seeking to innovate and societies seeking to affect change. Because individuals and organizations utilize design-thinking for different purposes, it has been described in a variety of ways. Researchers are also continuing to work on design-thinking to improve human lives. As a result, there are numerous definitions of design available on online sites, articles, blogs, and elsewhere. To find all possible definitions that could possibly describe a thorough search was conducted.

The purpose of design-thinking is expressed by Brown (2009), design-thinking leverages human capacities that are underutilized in more traditional problem solving practices. It is not only human-centered, it is also intensely human. Design-thinking is based on the human ability to be intuitive, recognize patterns, develop ideas with emotional meaning as well as functionality, and express them via mediums other than words or symbols. Nobody wants to operate a firm purely on emotion, intuition, and inspiration, but relying too heavily on logic and analysis can be just as disastrous.

Grots & Creuznacher (2016) mentioned that design-thinking assists in dealing with ambiguity, articulating the correct questions, and identifying and formulating possibilities and potentials. According to the authors, design-thinking provides suggestions on how to ask the proper questions to clients so that the true problem of the customers may be understood. It is difficult for designers to design for clients if they do not identify the correct problems.

According to Skaggs (2018), design-thinking is the use of observation, experience, and inquiry that allows designers to understand human needs and shape information to drive the creation of products and experiences that make human connections through aesthetics, need-finding, or creating meaning.

Micheli et al. (2019)'s definition of design-thinking, has attracted considerable interest from practitioners and academics alike, as it offers a novel approach to innovation and problem solving. However, there appear to be substantial differences between promoters and critics about its essential attributes, applicability, and outcomes.

Schallmo et al. (2018) carried out an extensive study and offered an additional definition of design-thinking: *the goal of the design-thinking methodology is to create original solutions to problems that already exist.* These solutions continually focus on user requirements and have a beneficial effect. Iterative and systematic processes characterize design-thinking. A diverse team employs methods during the design-thinking process.

The design team from IDEO U. Design Thinking Framework, Innovation and Methodology, (2023) presented a great definition of design-thinking: *design-thinking is a human-centered innovation strategy built on understanding client demands, rapid prototyping, and coming up with original ideas that will revolutionize how designers create goods, services, procedures, and organizations.* Instead of making hazardous bets based solely on historical data or relying on a hunch rather than proof, designers use design-thinking to base their conclusions on what clients desire.

From these definitions, it can be said that *design-thinking is a method for approaching complicated problems from the perspective of the user to improve people's lives.* Design-Thinking is a strategy for creative problem solving by prioritizing customers' requirements above everything else. It helps to engage a person in several opportunities, like experimenting and creating a prototype model, gathering feedback from customers, and redesigning products using innovative solutions.

In recent years, design-thinking has evolved and expanded beyond the realm of product design. It has been applied to various fields, including business, education, healthcare, and social innovation. Design-thinking is now seen as a valuable framework for solving complex problems and driving innovation in a wide range of contexts.

1.3 Advantages of Design-Thinking

Using design-thinking techniques in the workplace has various advantages. The biggest advantage is being able to identify issues that clients are experiencing. Design-thinking focuses on customer needs and implements processes based on those needs. Although design-thinking provides satisfaction for clients, it also provides benefits to designers. Tadevosyan, K (2023) explains some advantages of design-thinking, which we consider below:

1.3.1 Enhances User-Centric Solutions

Design-thinking enhances user-centric solutions by placing the user at the center of the design process. User-centered design (UCD) is a proactive strategy for coming up with novel ideas. Humans are the starting point, and answers that are specific to their needs are the finish line. Novel solutions are generated when the target audience is identified and solutions are created considering their perspective. UCD describes both the way that designers think and what they do. It all comes down to developing a strong sense of empathy for the people the designs are intended for.

The process of user-centered design is iterative, with four distinct phases involved in each iteration, as shown in Figure 1.2. Initially, as collaborative designers, attempt to comprehend the environment in which users might utilize a system. They then ascertain and describe user needs. The team then moves on to the design phase, where they develop solutions. Following this is the evaluation phase, where they review the evaluation results about the user's needs and context to determine the effectiveness of the design.

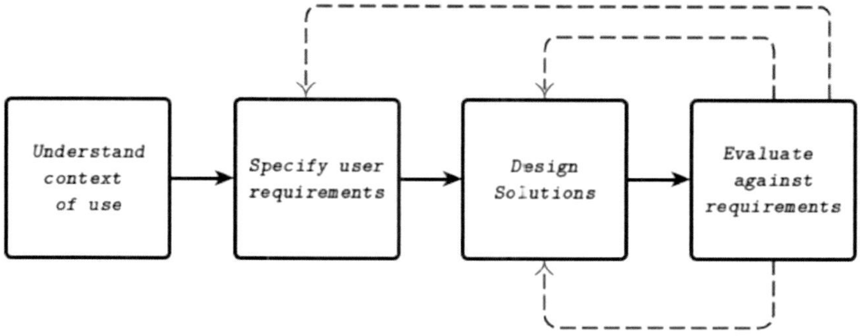

Figure 1.2: Four Phases of User-Centered Design

1.3.2 Encourages Innovation and Creative Thinking

Innovative thinking is encouraged by design-thinking, which promotes the investigation of novel concepts and creative solutions that might not otherwise be taken into account. Businesses can tackle issues and challenges from different angles, which leads to creative solutions that can differentiate them from rivals. Design-thinking can raise consumer happiness and loyalty by concentrating on their desires and experiences. Design-thinking also promotes experimentation and risk-taking due to its collaborative and iterative character, which can result in game-changing insights and new opportunities. Notably, while creativity and innovation are both crucial components of design-thinking, they have distinct functions and traits, as shown in Table 1.1.

Table 1.1: Innovation vs Creativity

Innovation	Creativity
The process of developing novel concepts, items, or procedures that have a big influence on the market or society is known as innovation.	The capacity to produce unique and imaginative notions, ideas, or designs is known as creativity.
The main objective is to apply fresh and improved answers to current issues or requirements.	Entails thinking creatively and investigating novel approaches to problem solving.
Entails taking original concepts and turning them into useful, practical products.	Creativity is the cornerstone of innovation because it offers the starting point for fresh, original solutions.
Brings about change and improvement, frequently takes teamwork, experimentation, and taking risks.	Techniques like mind mapping, lateral thinking, and brainstorming can assist in fostering creativity.

To put it briefly, innovation is the process of putting creative ideas into practice to create value, whereas creativity is the process of coming up with unique and imaginative concepts that can inspire innovation. Recognizing and taking advantage of unmet opportunities and needs, are both critical components of design-thinking. Design-thinking is a useful tool for companies trying to expand through innovation and creativity while remaining competitive.

1.3.3 Encourages Problem Reframing

Design-thinking enables businesses to reframe difficulties and see them from several angles, which promotes a deeper comprehension of the underlying problems and the discovery of more comprehensive solutions. It promotes problem reframing, which is the process of examining a problem from many aspects and viewpoints to generate novel ideas and opportunities. This strategy can assist companies in locating the root causes of their problems and resolving them more successfully. Businesses can come up with more original and creative solutions by rephrasing problems that may not have been obvious in the past. This procedure may produce ground-breaking concepts and fresh chances that will keep organizations one step ahead of the competition. In general, problem reframing is a significant benefit of design-thinking that can assist companies in resolving complicated issues and fostering growth.

1.3.4 Emphasizes Collaboration and Teamwork Towards Realistic Outcomes

Design-thinking encourages cross-functional cooperation and teamwork by bringing different viewpoints and specialties together to address complicated issues. As it entails bringing together people with various experiences, abilities, and viewpoints to work toward a similar objective, it places a strong emphasis on collaboration and teamwork. This strategy promotes candid communication, attentive listening, and empathy for other people's perspectives. Teams that collaborate well can come up with mordiverse ideas and viewpoints, which leads to more creative solutions. Additionally, the co-creation and iteration processes enable ongoing input and development, which may produce superior results. In general, design-thinking's key benefits of cooperation and teamwork can promote success, innovation, and creativity.

1.3.5 Focus on Rapid Prototyping and Testing

Design-thinking places a focus on rapidly testing and developing ideas, enabling firms to obtain feedback early on and make required adjustments before devoting a large amount of resources. To quickly iterate and refine ideas, design-thinking highlights the value of rapid prototyping and testing. To acquire feedback and insights, low-fidelity prototypes, such as sketches or mock-ups, must be created and tested with users. Teams can find potential problems and make the required corrections by testing frequently and early before devoting a lot of time and resources to a solution or final product. A mindset of experimentation and learning from failure is also promoted by rapid prototyping and testing, which results in more creative and efficient solutions. All things considered, this strategy enables quicker development cycles, higher user involvement, and ultimately, more successful results.

1.3.6 Coordinating Continuous Improvement

Design-thinking's iterative nature enables businesses to continuously learn from mistakes, modify ideas in response to user feedback, and make small but steady advancements over time. Design-thinking promotes a continuous improvement process that enables teams to develop their ideas over time through quick prototyping and testing. Teams may pinpoint problem areas and make the required changes to their prototypes by getting input from users and stakeholders. The outcome or solution will more likely satisfy the demands and expectations of the target market if an iterative approach is used to create it. The emphasis on continual improvement also encourages a culture of invention and creativity because teams are urged to experiment with fresh concepts and methods to produce more comprehensive results. This strategy may ultimately result in more efficient solutions that align with user requirements and preferences.

1.3.7 Enhances User Experience

Design-thinking assists in developing solutions that offer a more comprehensive user experience, increasing customer pleasure and loyalty. It empathizes with people and includes them in the design process. Design-thinking assists teams in developing solutions and products that are suited to the needs and preferences of the user by putting them at the center of the design process. A more intuitive and user-friendly experience is produced as a result, which may boost consumer happiness and loyalty. Teams can uncover problems and opportunities for improvement by soliciting user feedback throughout the design process, creating a more seamless and pleasurable user experience. In the end, this may result in greater usage and adoption of the product or solution as well as favorable word-of-mouth referrals. In general, design-thinking can assist teams in producing goods and solutions that resonate with their target market, resulting in greater outcomes and more comprehensive user experiences.

1.3.8 Reduces Risk

Design-thinking helps reduce the risk of creating solutions that do not fulfill user needs or expectations by including users early in the design process and receiving input through prototyping and testing. By enabling teams to test and iterate on their ideas before devoting substantial resources to development, design-thinking also helps to lower risk. Teams can find possible problems early in the process and make changes before releasing the finished product by performing user research and prototyping. In the long term, this can save time and money and stop people from leaving disappointing comments or reviews. Additionally, teams can lower the likelihood of developing a product or solution that falls short by ensuring that their solutions are in line with business objectives and user demands by including stakeholders and users throughout the design process.

1.3.9 Competitive Advantage

Design-thinking may help firms stand out from the competition by empowering them to develop distinctive and ground-breaking solutions that stand out in the marketplace. Teams can develop unique, user-centered solutions that set them apart from the competition by utilizing design-thinking. Teams may develop goods and services that stand out in the market and offer a distinctive value proposition by comprehending the wants and desires of their target customers. As a result, there is perhaps a rise in client loyalty, more sales, and a better reputation for the company. Design-thinking can also give businesses a long-term competitive advantage by assisting them in anticipating future requirements and staying ahead of industry trends.

1.3.10 Cultural Transformation

Adopting design-thinking can assist firms in developing a culture of creativity, collaboration, and ongoing learning, which will boost employee engagement and organizational success. Additionally, design-thinking can result in cultural change inside a company. Teams may eliminate silos and foster an innovative and creative culture through human-centered, cooperative problem solving. Increased retention, work satisfaction, and employee engagement may result from this. Additionally, design-thinking can assist businesses in becoming more flexible and agile, enabling them to react swiftly to shifting market circumstances and client demands. Overall, design-thinking can assist businesses in developing a culture of innovation and continual improvement, which is crucial for long-term success in the quickly shifting business environment of today.

1.4 Design-Thinking Goals

The main goal of design thinkers is to create goods, services, procedures, and strategies that meet people's requirements. They combine what is technologically possible and financially practical with what is desirable from the perspective of the client. Additionally, design-thinking gives non-designers many possibilities to use creative tools to address a wide range of issues and barriers. According to

Raju, K.S. (2022), the following are some crucial areas where design-thinking is helpful.

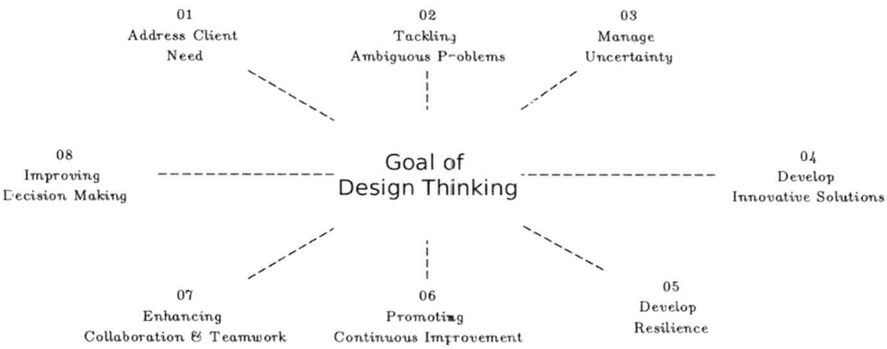

Figure 1.3: Goals of Design-Thinking Approach

1.4.1 Addressing Client Needs

Meeting consumer needs, and addressing preferences, and pain points is the primary goal of the design-thinking process. To understand the needs of their customers, design thinkers first interview them extensively and have discussions in groups. As a result of these interviews and discussions, problems are identified using the empathy and define phases of design-thinking. These phases will be discussed in the following chapters. Design-thinking can assist businesses in producing solutions that are suited to user requirements and preferences, resulting in greater customer loyalty and satisfaction.

1.4.2 Tackling Ambiguous Problems

Tackling ambiguous problems is another important goal in design-thinking as it allows for a more holistic and creative approach to problem solving. The state of having more than one conceivable meaning or interpretation is called ambiguity. When handling complicated and vague topics, ambiguity can be a source of confusion, frustration, and conflict. However, It also provides a chance to examine many viewpoints, come up with a variety of concepts, and gain new insights. Accepting uncertainty is a necessary component of the design-thinking process as opposed to attempting to eradicate it. Design-thinking is an iterative, non-linear approach that can address ambiguous challenges.

1.4.3 Managing Uncertainty

Uncertainty is the inability to foresee or forecast the results or repercussions of a choice or action. Particularly when working with dynamic and uncertain circumstances, it can be a cause of anxiety, doubt, and risk. Nevertheless, uncertainty can also be a source of knowledge, criticism, and development. Design-thinking embraces uncertainty and manages it by taking an open-minded approach to problem solving. Design-thinking recognizes uncertainty as a normal component of problem solving and aims to comprehend and effectively navigate it rather than trying to eradicate it.

Design-thinking, with its human-centered methodology, concentrates on developing an in-depth understanding of end-users' needs and behaviors. By revealing their preferences and pain points, this approach can assist in reducing uncertainty. With this knowledge, solutions can be created that are more likely to satisfy the needs of the intended audience and make more comprehensive decisions.

Furthermore, a culture of experimentation and iteration is fostered by design-thinking, enabling designers to test and improve their ideas to learn from mistakes and enhance solutions. Because iterative processes enable continuous improvement and adaptation based on feedback and new insights, they aid in the management of uncertainty.

1.4.4 Developing Innovative Solutions

Innovation is the capability to envision, create, implement, and scale new products, services, processes, or business models that provide value to customers. It can assist designers in gaining a competitive edge, resolving client issues, and producing value for their company and society. It can also assist designers in coming up with innovative and workable ideas that satisfy the requirements and expectations of their users.

1.4.5 Developing Resilience

The capacity to handle challenges and bounce back from failures is called resilience. Coping with rejection and failure can be a source of strength, adaptation, and growth. Resilience can, however, also lead to stress, tiredness, and burnout, particularly when coping with ongoing pressure and change. Developing resilience as part of the design thinking process involves embracing challenges, failures, and setbacks as opportunities for learning and growth rather than trying to avoid them. Failure is viewed as a chance for growth, success as a major accomplishment, and assistance as a resource. Resiliency within a team is built by using tools like feedback, reflection, and appreciation.

1.4.6 Promoting Continuous Improvement

Design-thinking encourages organizations to iterate and develop their solutions based on feedback and insights from users, which promotes continuous improvement. It emphasizes the value of prototyping and testing ideas to make quick changes and revisions. Organizations can find areas for development and implement the necessary adjustments by understanding users' requirements and empathizing with them. Collaboration and a diversity of viewpoints are also encouraged by design-thinking, which can result in creative ideas and solutions that develop and become more comprehensive over time.

1.4.7 Enhancing Collaboration and Teamwork

Design-thinking encourages organizations to incorporate a variety of viewpoints and areas of expertise throughout the design process, which improves collaboration and teamwork. It emphasizes the value of interdisciplinary cooperation by bringing together people from various backgrounds and academic fields to share their special ideas and talents. It uses techniques like empathy, ideation, prototyping, testing, and brainstorming that demand collaboration and feedback from teams. As teams collaborate continuously to hone and improve their solutions in response to user feedback and insights, this iterative process promotes cooperation and ongoing collaboration. In general, design-thinking encourages a collaborative and inclusive problem solving approach, improving teamwork and enabling organizations to tap into the collective intelligence and creativity of their teams.

1.4.8 Improving Decision Making

Organizations may make more comprehensive, informed and successful decisions based on user insights and feedback giving design-thinking's structured and methodical approach to problem solving. Design-thinking can encourage teams to collect and evaluate data, understand stakeholders, and take into account various points of view (POV) before making a choice, which can enhance decision making. By using this method, judgments can be made that are more informed, more sensible, and more in line with the requirements of the concerned individuals. A more equitable and inclusive conclusion can be achieved by using design-thinking to assist teams in recognizing and addressing potential biases that perhaps influence their decision making. Design-thinking can assist teams in making decisions, learning from them, and enhancing their procedures over time by encouraging an environment of experimentation and iteration.

1.5 Applications of Design-Thinking

Design-thinking is used to address complicated problems and spur creativity in a variety of disciplines, including sports, education, research, and industry (Tselepis & Lavelle, 2020). The following are some typical uses of design-thinking:

1.5.1 Business Strategy and Innovation

Application of design-thinking can lead to the creation of new business models, the discovery of market opportunities, and organizational innovation. Giving decision making and problem solving a formal framework also aids company strategy and innovation. It aids businesses in identifying market opportunities, learning about the needs and goals of their clients, and coming up with innovative solutions. The benefit of design-thinking is that it entails conducting user research, empathizing with the target audience, and learning about their habits and preferences. This aids companies in better comprehending the problems that their clients have and developing goods and services that efficiently address those problems.

A collaborative and iterative approach to problem solving is also encouraged by design-thinking. It promotes collaboration, idea sharing, and experimentation across cross-functional teams, as well as the use of various approaches. As a result, the company might develop new business models or strategies that set them apart from rivals and promote an innovative culture within the company. Additionally, design-thinking emphasizes early idea testing and prototyping. This enables companies to obtain consumer input and alter their operations depending on their observations. Businesses can produce unique solutions that have a higher chance of becoming successful in the market by iterating and improving their concepts over time.

In general, design-thinking assists businesses in creating a customer-centric strategy and innovation process. They can use it to find unmet requirements, develop useful solutions, and maintain their competitive edge in a market that is undergoing rapid change.

1.5.2 Product and Service Design

Design-thinking is a methodical way of analyzing consumer demands, developing ideas, and prototyping solutions, which aids in the creation of products and services. It primarily focuses on user-centered products and services by understanding the needs and preferences of the target audience. Through brainstorming sessions, design-thinking pushes firms to produce a wide range of ideas. This creative process aids in the generation of original and priceless ideas for the design of goods and services. Businesses may quickly obtain customer feedback and make essential modifications by producing low-fidelity prototypes. To ensure that the final design fulfills user expectations, this iterative method enables quick trial and refinement of product or service concepts. As a result, it produces a more user-centric and effective final product or service.

Finally and above all, design-thinking encourages cooperation across teams made up of designers, engineers, marketers, and business strategists. Businesses can develop comprehensive, well-rounded designs that take into account several factors, such as usability, feasibility, and marketability, by enlisting the assistance of numerous viewpoints and experts.

1.5.3 Education

Students' creativity, problem solving skills, and critical thinking are developed in educational institutions that use design-thinking. Additionally, it can be applied to improve learning for both teachers and students. Teachers obtain an opportunity to empathize with children and comprehend their individual needs, difficulties, and motivations through design-thinking. Educators can discover ways to better support students' learning processes by doing user research and monitoring them in their learning settings. Design-thinking also encourages the development of fun and dynamic learning experiences. Teachers can improve learning for students by introducing features like gamification, practical exercises, and real-world applications.

Design-thinking promotes an iterative way of teaching in which teachers regularly solicit student feedback and revise their lesson plans or curriculum. This enables teachers to modify their strategy in response to the wants and preferences of their students, which enhances the learning process. Additionally, design-thinking imparts important problem solving abilities to students. Teachers can support children in the development of critical thinking, creativity, and resilience by encouraging them to identify problems or obstacles, generate ideas, prototype solutions, and test them out.

Design-thinking places a strong emphasis on teamwork and collaboration, which are crucial abilities for students to develop. Teachers can encourage students to cooperate, exchange ideas, and learn from one another by integrating group projects and collaborative activities into the curriculum.

1.5.4 Healthcare

To improve the patient experience and the provision of healthcare services, design-thinking can also be employed in the healthcare industry. The needs, preferences, and experiences of patients are given priority in a patient-centered approach to healthcare. Healthcare professionals can build services and procedures that match patients' unique requirements and enhance their overall experience by understanding and empathizing with them. Additionally, design-thinking pushes healthcare professionals to locate probable sources of medical errors and deal with them. It enhances patient safety by applying design principles to healthcare operations, such as developing simple and user-friendly interfaces for electronic medical records or developing prescription administration systems with low error rates.

Healthcare professionals are encouraged to handle complicated challenges creatively and ingeniously by using design-thinking. Design-thinking can assist in creating novel solutions that enhance patient care by applying design principles to healthcare difficulties like creating new medical devices or creating new care delivery models. Iterative approaches to problem solving and improvement are encouraged by design-thinking. Design-thinking may support ongoing improvements in the effectiveness and quality of healthcare delivery by soliciting feedback from patients and healthcare professionals and making iterative adjustments to healthcare services and systems.

1.5.5 Environmental Sustainability

Environmental sustainability can also benefit from the application of design-thinking to handle difficult environmental issues and produce original solutions. Environmental concerns can be recognized and examined using design-thinking techniques, which can assist people in understanding their underlying causes and possible remedies. This is the foundation upon which design-thinking develops solutions that are engaging, user-friendly, and consistent with people's values and behaviors. Increased adoption and long-term viability of environmentally friendly practices and technologies may result from this.

Design-thinking makes it simple to comprehend the intricate interactions between social, economic, and environmental aspects, and to create solutions that take these interdependencies into account. To obtain input and improve designs may entail developing sustainable product or service prototypes and testing them in actual environments. To increase the effectiveness and sustainability of solutions, it is necessary to regularly assess effects, collect feedback, and make iterative modifications.

1.5.6 User Experience (UX) Design

Design-thinking focuses on user demands and behaviors to enhance the usability and overall experience of digital interfaces, websites, and applications. Understanding people's needs, wants, and pain areas is a key component of design-thinking. This empathic approach enables UX designers to learn about the experiences of people and create solutions that solve their issues.

The user is central to the process of design-thinking. To fully comprehend consumers and their context, tools like personas, user journey mapping, and user research are used. The final design will conform to consumere expectations and objectives with this user-centric approach. The iterative approach of design-thinking encourages designers to continuously test and improve their concepts in light of user feedback. This strategy enables UX designers to quickly spot and address usability problems, thereby improving the user experience.

1.5.7 Social Innovation

Design-thinking can also be applied to social innovation, which involves addressing complex social issues and creating positive change in society. Design-thinking starts by empathizing with people affected by a social issue. By deeply understanding their needs, challenges, and aspirations, insights into the root causes of the problem can be gained, and opportunities identified for innovative solutions. Design-thinking encourages collaboration among stakeholders, including community members, experts, policymakers, and organizations. By involving diverse perspectives and expertise, an optimal solution can be co-created that is holistic, inclusive, and sustainable. Design-thinking involves generating a wide range of ideas and rapidly prototyping them. This approach allows social innovators to explore different approaches and test their viability before investing significant resources. Prototyping also helps in gathering feedback from users and refining the solutions based on their input.

Design-thinking takes a systems-level approach to social innovation. It is important to consider the interconnectedness of various factors and stakeholders involved in a social issue. By understanding the broader context and interdependencies, solutions can be developed that address the underlying causes and have a more significant impact. Similar to UX design, design-thinking in social innovation focuses on creating solutions that are not only effective but also meaningful and desirable for the people they aim to serve. By putting the needs and aspirations of the target population at the center, solutions can be created that resonate with them and drive positive change.

1.5.8 Government and Public Policy

Applying human-centered design principles and methods to the creation and execution of policies and programs is referred to as government and public policy in design-thinking. To develop creative, innovative, and responsive policies that better address the community's needs and concerns, entails understanding experiences of citizens, engaging diverse stakeholders, testing ideas in real-world settings, and fostering a culture of creativity and innovation.

By applying design-thinking principles to government and public policy, policymakers can create policies and services that are more citizen-centric, collaborative, evidence-based, and effective. This can lead to improved public services, increased citizen engagement, and better outcomes for society.

These are just a few examples, however, design-thinking can be applied in almost any industry or domain where there is a need for creative problem solving and innovation.

1.6 Conclusion

This chapter provides an overview of various design-thinking approaches. The definition of design-thinking and its history were initially discussed. The benefits, purpose, and along with application of design-thinking across the various fields have been considered.

References

Alexander, C. 1964. Notes on the synthesis of form (Vol. 5). Harvard University Press.

Archer, L. 1965. Systematic method for designers. Council of Industrial Design. Retrieved from https://books.google.co.in/books?id=3sG7nQAACAAJ.

Archer, L.B. 1968. The structure of design processes (Unpublished doctoral dissertation). Royal College of Art.

Asimow, M. 1962. Introduction to design. (No Title).

Brown, T. 2009. Change by Design: How Design Thinking Transforms Organizations and Inspires Innovation. HarperCollins. Retrieved from https://books.google.co.in/books?id=x7PjWyVUoVAC.

Buchanan, R. 1992. Wicked problems in design thinking. Design issues. 8(2): 5–21.

Council, D. 2004. Double diamonds. london: UK. https://www.designcouncil.org.uk/our-resources/the-double-diamond/. (Accessed: Accessed: January 26, 2023).

Cross, N. 1982. Designerly ways of knowing. Design studies. 3(4): 221–227.

Dam, R.F. and Siang, T.U. 2022. The history of design thinking. https://www.interaction-design.org/literature/article/design-thinking-get-a-quick-overview-of-the-history. (Accessed: July 2, 2023).

Elmansy, R. 2021. The double diamond design thinking process and how to use it—designorate. https://www.designorate.com/the-double-diamond-design-thinking-process-and-how-to-use-it/. (Accessed: December 31, 2023)

Gordon, W. 1961. Synectics: The Development of Creative Capacity. Harper & Row.

Grots, A. and Creuznacher, I. 2016. Design thinking: Process or culture? a method for organizational change. Design Thinking for Innovation: Research and Practice. 183–191.

IdeaKeep. 2018. Design thinking: state of things. https://medium.com/@ideakeep/design-thinking-state-of-things-2e2359b9cc24. (Accessed: June 20, 2023)

IDEO U. Design Thinking Framework, Innovation and Methodology, 2023. Design thinking. https://www.ideou.com/pages/design-thinking. (Accessed: June 30, 2023)

Jones, J.C. and Thornley, D.G. 1963. Conference on design methods.

Lawson, B. 2006. How Designers Think: The Design Process Demystified. Routledge.

Lewis, C. and Rieman, J. 1993. Task-centered user interface design. A practical introduction.

McKim, R. 1972. Experiences in Visual Thinking. RH McKim Brooks/Cole.

Micheli, P., Wilner, S.J., Bhatti, S.H., Mura, M. and Beverland, M.B. 2019. Doing design thinking: conceptual review, synthesis, and research agenda. Journal of Product Innovation Management. 36(2): 124–148.

Osborn, A.F. 1963. Applied Imagination: Principles and Procedures of Creative Problem-solving. Charles Scribner's.

Raju, K.S. 2022. What is design thinking and why is it important? https://www.mygreatlearning.com/blog/importance-of-design-thinking/#history-of-design-thinking. (Accessed: July 01, 2023).

Renard, H. 2014. Cultivating design thinking in students through material inquiry. International Journal of Teaching and Learning in Higher Education. 26(3): 414–424.

Rowe, P.G. 1991. Design thinking. MIT press.

Schallmo, D., Williams, C.A. and Lang, K. 2018. An integrated design thinking approach-literature review, basic principles and roadmap for design thinking. *In*: Ispim innovation symposium. 1–18.

Simon, H.A. 1969. The sciences of the artificial. by herbert a. simon. MIT Press.

Skaggs, P. 2018. Design thinking: Empathy through observation, experience, and inquiry. *In*: Society for Information Technology and Teacher Education International Conference. 1168–1172.

Tadevosyan, K . 2023. 10 benefits of using design thinking for innovation. https://slash.co/articles/10-benefits-of-using-design-thinking-for-innovation/. (Accessed: August 20, 2023).

Tselepis, T.J. and Lavelle, C.A. 2020. Design thinking in entrepreneurship education: understanding framing and placements of problems. Acta Commercii. 20(1): 1–8.

University, L. 2021. 8 types of designers you could be. https://lesley.edu/article/8-types-of-designers-you-could-be. (Accessed: June 26, 2023).

Van Doren, H. 1954. Industrial design: a practical guide to product design and development. McGraw-Hill. Retrieved from https://books.google .co.in/ books?id=CzVQAAAAMAAJ.

Walker, R. 2003. The guts of a new machine. the new york times. https://www. nytimes.com/2003/11/30/magazine/the-guts-of-a-new-machine.html. (Accessed: Accessed: January 24, 2024).

Chapter 2

Principles of Design-Thinking

Design-thinking is a human-centered method for creative problem-framing and problem solving, as has been previously mentioned. It entails more than just developing creative ideas. It is based on several significant principles that offer a guiding framework and a set of values to guide decision making. These principles support designers in maintaining their attention on the aims, goals, and intended effects of a project, ensuring that their solutions are efficient, significant, and user-centered.

Design-thinking helps carefully consider the requirements and viewpoints of users, stakeholders, and the larger context in which a problem is present. This makes it more likely that the produced solutions will be applicable, and significant, and handle the underlying causes of the issue. Design-thinking principles also foster innovation and creativity by encouraging designers to think creatively, challenge assumptions, and weigh alternative solutions. It encourages an experimental and iterative approach continuously learns, adjusts, and improves ideas in accordance with inputs and insights gleaned from the design process.

Meinel, Christoph and Leifer, Larry (2011) of the Hasso Plattner Institute of Design at Stanford University (commonly known as d.school) identified four rules of design-thinking. These principles highlight the essential components that make design-thinking products both aesthetically pleasing and functional. This chapter discusses the following topics:

- Human Rule
- Ambiguity Rule
- Redesign Rule
- Tangibility Rule

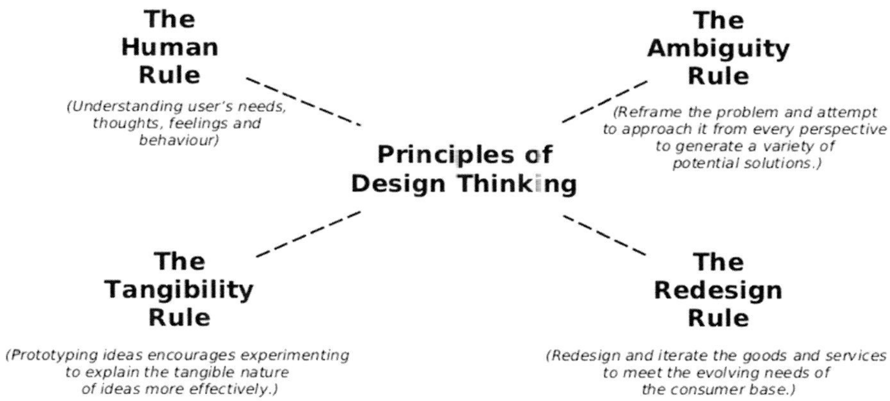

Figure 2.1: Principles of Design-Thinking

2.1 Human Rule

According to the human rule, companies can benefit greatly from developing goods and services with the end customer in mind and acknowledging the human element in all technologists. The needs, behaviors, and thought processes of the user must be understood by the design team. They ought to apply this information to come up with actual solutions to genuine issues. The Human-Centered Design principle is known as the "human rule" in design-thinking. Instead of imposing preconceived ideas or assumptions, it emphasizes building solutions that address the needs, desires, and behaviors of users. It entails comprehending and sharing the viewpoints, needs, and experiences of the individuals who will be impacted by the design. This principle acknowledges that the ultimate objective of design is to enhance the human experience and produce significant answers to demanding issues and challenges. Many kinds of people need to be considered in design-thinking (Dunne & Martin, 2006).

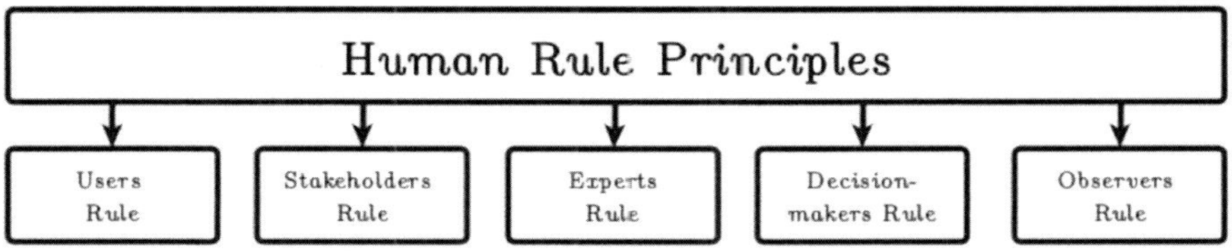

Figure 2.2: Types of Human Rule

2.1.1 End Users

End Users are the individuals who will directly interact with the designed thinking products. Understanding their needs, desires, and behaviors is crucial to creating a user-friendly and effective solution. Users are important in design-thinking because they are the ultimate beneficiaries, users, of the product or service being designed. Design-thinking is a human-centered approach that focuses on understanding and addressing the needs, desires, and pain points of theses users.

By involving users in all phases of the design process, a great deal of insight can be gained into their preferences, actions, and motivations. This helps to create solutions that actually meet the needs of customers and provide a pleasurable user experience. Design-thinking places a strong emphasis on understanding user. To completely understand perspectives, emotions, and challenges, designers try to put themselves in their client's shoes. This empathy allows for the creation of intuitive, significant, and impactful solutions.

Feedback can be obtained to validate hypotheses and make iterative improvements to designs by involving users in the design process through techniques such as user research, interviews, and usability testing. Because of this iterative process, the final products or services are tailored to the needs and preferences of the customers.

Finally, by prioritizing users in the design-thinking process, solutions can be created that are not only aesthetically pleasing but also practical, usable, and enjoyable for those for whom they are intended. Several types of people collaborate with designers to create products for customers, including *stakeholders, experts, decision-makers, and observers.*

2.1.2 Stakeholders

Stakeholders are crucial in design-thinking as they have a vested stake in the success of the product or service being designed. Individuals or groups such as investors, executives, managers, employees, and customers are examples of stakeholders (Dam, R. F and Siang, T Y , 2022). Designers can more comprehensively understand stakeholders' perspectives, aspirations, and requirements by involving them in the design process. This ensures that the final solution is in line with overall business goals and meets the needs of all stakeholders.

Stakeholders frequently provide useful insights and knowledge that can help with the design process. They are likely familiar with market trends, industry laws, and customer preferences that can help guide design decisions. Designers can tap into this collective expertise and create better-informed design decisions. Stakeholders can also contribute comments and validation during the design process. Their feedback can assist designers in refining and improving their concepts, ensuring that the finished product or service.

Involving stakeholders in the design process also fosters a sense of ownership and buy-in. Stakeholders are more inclined to support and advocate for the final solution when they feel heard and included in the decision making process. This can lead to a more successful deployment of the proposed product or service. Overall, stakeholders are crucial in design-thinking because their participation assists designers in developing solutions that correspond with company objectives, address user demands, and win support from relevant persons or organizations.

2.1.3 Experts

Experts are vital in design-thinking because they provide specialized knowledge and skills for the design process. They have comprehensive expertise in their subject or sector, which can bring useful insights and views that inspire design decisions. Experts assist designers in gaining knowledge of the situation at hand by providing insights into underlying issues, context, and restrictions. Their knowledge can assist designers in identifying viable solutions and evaluating feasibility, and desirability.

Experts can also act as mentors or advisers, leading designers through the design process and providing comments and direction along the way. They can provide useful feedback during brainstorming sessions, assist in the refinement of ideas, and make suggestions for improvement. Experts are also essential in validating and testing design solutions. Their knowledge enables them to evaluate a solution's effectiveness and usability, finding any potential flaws or opportunities for development. This contributes to the final design meeting the needs and expectations of users.

Furthermore, experts can contribute to a design solution's general credibility and validity. Their approval or support can offer legitimacy to the design process and boost confidence in the final result. Experts contribute essential information, insights, direction, and validation to the design-thinking process as a whole. Their knowledge improves the quality and efficacy of design solutions, allowing designers to build more meaningful and impactful solutions.

2.1.4 Decision-Makers

Decision-makers are important in design-thinking because they have the authority and responsibility to make final decisions regarding design solutions. They play a crucial role in determining which ideas and solutions will be implemented and have the power to allocate resources and support for the design process. Decision-makers provide the necessary support and buy-in for design projects. Their involvement and endorsement help secure the necessary resources, budget, and support from stakeholders and higher-level management. Without their support, it can be challenging to implement and execute design solutions effectively.

Furthermore, decision-makers have a broader perspective and understanding of the organization's goals, objectives, and constraints. They can provide valuable insights into the strategic direction and priorities of the organization, ensuring that design solutions align with overall goals and objectives. Decision-makers also have the authority to make trade-offs and prioritize different design options. They can weigh the potential benefits and risks of different solutions and make informed decisions based on their understanding of the organization's needs and constraints.

In addition, decision-makers can help drive organizational change and the adoption of design-thinking principles. Their support and commitment to the design process can influence the culture and mindset within the organization, promoting a more user-centered and innovative approach to problem solving.

Overall, decision-makers are important in design-thinking because they provide the necessary support, resources, and strategic guidance for design projects. Their involvement ensures that design solutions align with organizational goals and priorities and helps drive the adoption of design-thinking principles within the organization.

2.1.5 Observers

These are individuals who may not directly interact with the design solution but can provide valuable feedback and insights. Observers can be researchers, market analysts, or other professionals who can offer a different perspective on the design challenge. Considering the needs, desires, and behaviors of these different categories of people ensures that the design solution is inclusive, effective, and meets expectations of all stakeholders. Observers are important in design-thinking because they provide an external perspective and fresh insights into the design process. They are typically individuals who are not directly involved in the design project but have relevant expertise or knowledge.

Observers can bring a different set of skills, experiences, and perspectives to the table. They can offer valuable feedback, suggestions, and alternative viewpoints that may not have been considered by the design team. This can help challenge assumptions, uncover blind spots, and generate new ideas. By observing the design process, observers can also provide objective and unbiased feedback. They can identify potential flaws or weaknesses in the design solutions and offer constructive criticism. This feedback can be invaluable in refining and improving the design solutions before implementation.

Furthermore, observers can act as advocates for end-users or stakeholders. They can represent their interests and needs throughout the design process, ensuring that the final solutions are user-centered and meet their requirements.

Observers can also play a role in facilitating collaboration and communication within the design team. They can help bridge gaps between different team members, facilitate discussions, and ensure that all voices are heard. Overall, observers bring an external perspective, expertise, and unbiased feedback to the design-thinking process. Their involvement can help challenge assumptions, generate new ideas, improve the quality of the design solutions, and ensure that the end user's needs are met.

2.2 Ambiguity Rule

The ambiguity rule refers to the fact that ambiguity cannot be eliminated or oversimplified as it is an unavoidable reality. This rule emphasizes the value of testing the boundaries of one's knowledge to develop new perspectives. In short, the ambiguity rule encourages considering all potential solutions to a dilemma. Additionally, this guideline promotes an open-minded attitude to the design process and a level of comfort with all solutions not being immediately available. Through idea-testing and prototyping the ambiguity rule encourages experimentation, iteration, and learning. Designers can gain new perspectives, come across unexpected opportunities, and develop ground-breaking solutions that take into account the complexity and uncertainty of real-world issues by embracing ambiguity (Abell & DeVore, 2017). In design-thinking, various kinds of ambiguity can occur:

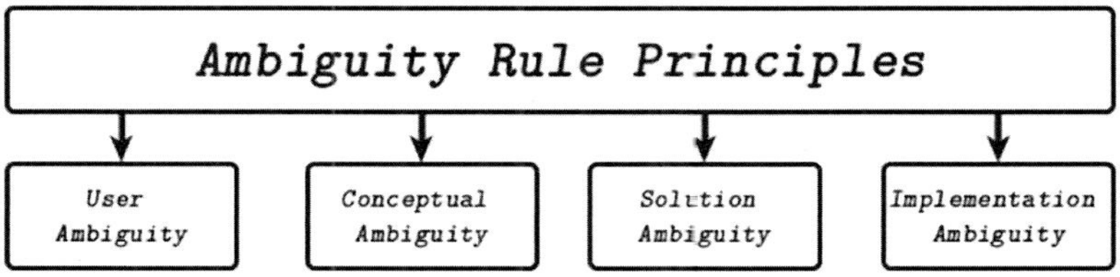

Figure 2.3: Ambiguity Rule

2.2.1 User Ambiguity

This refers to uncertainty or lack of understanding about the needs, preferences, and behaviors of the users or stakeholders involved in the design process. Designers may need to gather more information, conduct research, or engage in user testing to gain a clearer understanding of user needs and preferences. It is important in design-thinking to allow for a more open and exploratory approach to understanding the needs and preferences of users. When there is ambiguity concerning the user, designers are encouraged to question assumptions and gather more diverse perspectives.

By embracing user ambiguity, designers can avoid making assumptions or stereotyping users based on limited information. They are encouraged to conduct research, engage in empathy-building activities, and gather data from a wide range of sources to gain a deeper understanding of the user's context, needs, and desires. User ambiguity also fosters creativity and innovation in the design process. When designers are not constrained by preconceived notions about the user, they are more likely to think outside the box and come up with novel solutions. This can lead to the development of more impactful and user-centered designs.

Additionally, user ambiguity allows for flexibility and adaptability in the design process. As new information and insights about the user emerge, designers can iterate and refine their designs to better meet their needs. This iterative approach helps designers stay responsive to changing user requirements and market dynamics.

Finally, embracing user ambiguity can lead to more inclusive and accessible designs. By recognizing that users are diverse and have different backgrounds, abilities, and preferences, designers can create solutions that cater to a wider range of users. This helps ensure that no one is left behind and that the design solutions are truly inclusive.

2.2.2 Conceptual Ambiguity

This refers to a lack of clarity or understanding about the problem or design challenge itself. It may involve uncertainty about the goals, objectives, or requirements of the project, making it difficult to determine a strong approach or solution. Conceptual ambiguity is important in design-thinking because it allows for a more flexible and creative exploration of ideas and concepts. When there is ambiguity in the conceptualization of a problem or solution, designers are encouraged to explore multiple interpretations and possibilities.

By embracing conceptual ambiguity, designers can avoid getting stuck in rigid or narrow thinking. They can challenge conventional ideas and assumptions, which can lead to innovative and groundbreaking solutions. This openness to ambiguity promotes a mindset of curiosity and exploration, enabling designers to think outside the box and come up with fresh perspectives. Conceptual ambiguity also encourages collaboration and diverse thinking. When the concept is ambiguous, designers are more likely to seek input and feedback from others. This can lead to a more inclusive and diverse range of ideas, as different individuals bring unique perspectives and experiences to the table. By embracing conceptual ambiguity, designers foster an environment that values diverse voices and promotes collective problem solving.

Furthermore, conceptual ambiguity allows for adaptability and iteration in the design process. As new insights and understandings emerge, designers can refine and iterate their concepts to more comprehensively address the problem or meet user needs. This iterative approach helps designers stay responsive to changing requirements and market dynamics. Therefore, conceptual ambiguity promotes empathy and user-centeredness in design-thinking. When the concept is ambiguous, designers are encouraged to deeply understand the needs, desires, and contexts of users. They engage in research, empathy-building activities, and user-testing to gather insights and ensure that their concepts are truly user-centered.

2.2.3 Solution Ambiguity

This refers to multiple possible solutions or approaches to given problem, without clarity on which is most effective or appropriate. Designers may need to explore and experiment with different options before settling on a final solution. The ambiguity rule in design-thinking refers to embracing and exploring uncertainty and ambiguity during the design process. It encourages designers to not rush to find a single solution or answer right away but instead to embrace multiple possibilities and ideas.

The ambiguity rule recognizes that in complex design challenges, there may not be a clear-cut or obvious solution from the beginning. By allowing for ambiguity, designers can explore different perspectives, challenge assumptions, and generate a wide range of potential solutions. It is important in design-thinking to allow for a more open and exploratory approach to finding solutions to a problem. When there is ambiguity in the definition of a solution, designers are encouraged to consider a wide range of possibilities and alternatives.

By embracing solution ambiguity, designers can avoid prematurely settling on a single solution and instead engage in a more iterative and adaptive process. They can explore different approaches, experiment with various ideas, and test multiple solutions to determine the most effective one.

Solution ambiguity also encourages designers to challenge assumptions and think critically about the problem they are trying to solve. It prompts them to question established norms and seek unconventional solutions that may not have been considered otherwise. This mindset of exploration and experimentation can lead to breakthrough innovations and unexpected outcomes.

Furthermore, solution ambiguity promotes collaboration and collective problem solving. When the solution is ambiguous, designers are more likely to seek input and feedback from others, including users, stakeholders, and experts in different fields. This collaborative approach brings diverse perspectives and expertise into the design process, leading to more robust and well-rounded solutions.

Additionally, solution ambiguity allows for adaptability and responsiveness to changing needs and circumstances. As designers gather new insights and feedback, they can refine and iterate their solutions to more comprehensively address the problem or meet user needs. This iterative approach ensures that the final solution is well suited to the specific context and requirements. Finally, solution ambiguity encourages designers to prioritize user-centeredness and empathy. When the solution is ambiguous, designers are prompted to deeply understand the needs, preferences, and behaviors of the users. They engage in user-research, testing, and feedback collection to ensure that the final solution is user-centric and provides a meaningful and satisfying experience.

2.2.4 Implementation Ambiguity

This type of ambiguity arises when there are uncertainties or challenges related to the implementation or execution of a design solution. It may involve technical constraints, resource limitations, or logistical issues that need to be addressed to bring the design to life.

Implementation ambiguity is important in design-thinking because it allows for flexibility and adaptability during the implementation phase of a solution. When there is ambiguity in how a solution will be implemented, designers are encouraged to consider different approaches and methods, leading to more creative and effective solutions.

By embracing implementation ambiguity, designers can avoid rigid and predetermined plans and instead be open to new ideas and possibilities. They can experiment with different strategies, techniques, and tools to find the most suitable way to bring their solution to life. This flexibility enables designers to adapt and respond to unexpected challenges or changes in the environment.

Implementation ambiguity also promotes collaboration and collective problem solving during the implementation process. When there is ambiguity in the implementation, designers are more likely to seek input and feedback from various stakeholders, including users, experts, and team members. This collaborative approach ensures that different perspectives are considered, leading to a more comprehensive and well-rounded implementation plan.

Furthermore, implementation ambiguity encourages designers to iterate and refine their implementation approach based on feedback and insights gathered during the process. They can continuously improve and adjust their methods to more comprehensively align with user needs and preferences. This iterative approach increases the chances of success and enhances the overall user experience.

Additionally, implementation ambiguity allows for experimentation and learning. Designers can try out different prototypes or versions of their solutions, gather feedback, and make adjustments accordingly. This trial-and-error process helps designers identify potential issues or areas for improvement early on, reducing the risk of failure in the final implementation.

Lastly, implementation ambiguity encourages designers to consider the feasibility and practicality of their solutions. When there is ambiguity in how a solution will be implemented, designers are prompted to think critically about the resources, constraints, and limitations that may affect the implementation process. This consideration ensures that the final solution is realistic and achievable within the given context.

2.3 Redesign Rule

Even though technology and social circumstances change, basic human needs remain constant, therefore, designers always greatly benefit from taking them into account when creating products. When designers redesign, they only change the means of solving the problem. In design-thinking, several kinds of redesigns can be applied to various aspects of a product or service. These redesigns aim to improve the user experience, functionality, and overall value of the design. Here are some common types of redesigns in design-thinking.

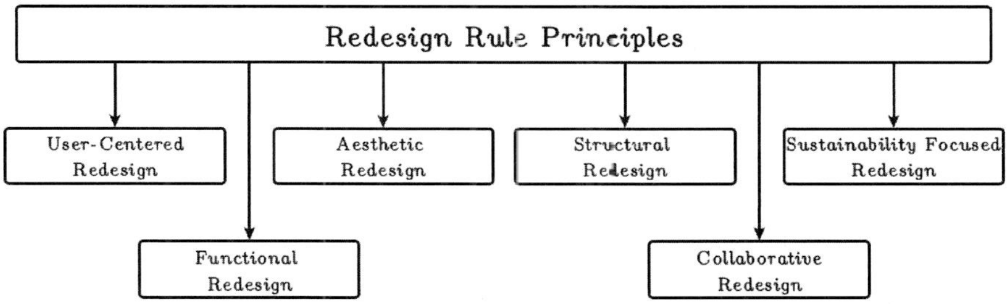

Figure 2.4: Redesign Rule

2.3.1 User-Centered Redesign

This type of redesign focuses on improving the design based on user needs and preferences. It involves gathering insights from users through research, observation, and feedback, and then incorporating these insights into the design to create a more user-friendly and intuitive experience. User-centered redesign is an approach to improving a product or system that focuses on the needs, preferences, and behaviors of end users. It involves gathering insights and feedback from users through various research methods, such as interviews, surveys, and usability testing.

The process begins by understanding the goals and tasks of users, as well as their pain points and frustrations with the current design. This information is used to inform the redesign process, ensuring that the new design addresses user needs and provides a more comprehensive user experience.

User-centered redesign typically involves iterative design cycles, where prototypes are created and tested with users. Feedback from users is collected and incorporated into subsequent iterations, gradually refining the design to better meet user requirements.

A new mobile app for online meal ordering is an illustration of user-centered redesign. The company learns through user feedback that the app is challenging to use and doesn't provide sufficient personalization. The company decides to go through a user-centered redesign approach to address the problem. They carry out user research to understand the requirements and preferences of their intended market. They produce fresh wireframes and prototypes based on this research that include user feedback and provide greater customization possibilities.

The ultimate goal of user-centered redesign is to create a product or system that is intuitive, efficient, and enjoyable to use. By involving users throughout the design process, the likelihood of creating a successful and user-friendly solution is greatly increased.

2.3.2 Functional Redesign

A functional redesign aims to enhance the functionality and performance of a design. It involves analyzing the existing design's features and capabilities and identifying areas for improvement or optimization. This type of redesign often consists of streamlining processes, reducing complexity, and enhancing efficiency.

An example of functional redesign using design-thinking could be the redesign of a kitchen appliance, such as a blender. Through the design-thinking process, the team identifies pain points and areas for improvement, such as difficulty in cleaning the blades or limited functionality.

The team can then ideate and prototype potential solutions, such as detachable blades for easier cleaning or additional features like a food processor attachment. These prototypes should be tested with real users to gather feedback and refine the design.

The final product would be a redesigned blender that not only functions comprehensively but also provides a better experience, resulting in increased customer satisfaction and loyalty.

2.3.3 Aesthetic Redesign

Aesthetic redesign focuses on improving the visual appeal and aesthetics of a design. It involves actions such as updating the color scheme, typography, layout, and overall visual elements to create a more visually pleasing and engaging format. An aesthetic redesign can also involve rebranding or refreshing a design to align with current trends or the preferences of a target audience.

Consider a business that offers handmade jewelry online. Although the website is useful and simple to use, the business is aware that it lacks a distinctive or memorable visual identity that distinguishes it from rivals. The business decided to go through an aesthetic makeover process to address this problem. They investigate the most recent design trends and get ideas from various jewelry-related websites and brands. They develop fresh mood boards and design ideas based on this study that feature original fonts, color schemes, and imagery.

The success of a product or service can be significantly impacted by aesthetic redesign, which is crucial in design-thinking (Tuusa, S, 2018). A product or service's aesthetics have a big impact on how customers perceive and use it. Customer happiness, brand loyalty, and sales can all be raised by a product or service's attractive and enticing design. A product or service's reputation can suffer if it has a poor or outdated design that turns away customers. Consumers frequently gravitate towards goods and services with a contemporary and eye-catching design, therefore, redesigning for aesthetic purposes is essential for remaining competitive in the market.

2.3.4 Structural Redesign

Structural redesign involves rethinking and modifying the underlying structure or architecture of a design. It aims to address any inherent flaws or limitations in the design's structure and make it more robust, flexible, and scalable. This type of redesign often requires a deep understanding of the design's technical aspects and may involve significant changes to the design's framework.

Using design-thinking, the redesign of a car dashboard can be considered as an illustration of structural redesign. Previously, it was challenging for drivers to operate the many operations of their vehicles because the dashboard was cluttered with numerous buttons, knobs, and dials. Structural redesign allows the automakers to simplify and streamline the dashboard, utilizing touchscreens and speech recognition technology to make it easier for drivers to access and use the car's amenities.

Design-thinking calls for structural redesign to increase a product or service's usability, functionality, and effectiveness. It entails reevaluating and rearranging a product's or service's fundamental design to more comprehensively fulfill user needs and handle any potential problems or hurdles.

Without structural redesign, products and services may become obsolete, challenging to use, or ineffective, which would lower consumer satisfaction and market competitiveness. Companies can enhance their products and services, remain ahead of the competition, and more comprehensively serve their consumers by applying design-thinking to identify structural redesign opportunities.

2.3.5 Collaborative Redesign

Collaborative redesign encompasses multiple users, such as designers, engineers, marketers, and end-users, in the redesign process. It emphasizes collaboration, brainstorming, and iterative prototyping to generate ideas and solutions that can address a wide range of perspectives and requirements.

An example of collaborative redesign in design-thinking is a company that wants to improve the user experience of its mobile app. The company would gather a diverse group of stakeholders, including app users, designers, developers, and customer service representatives, to participate in a design-thinking workshop. During the workshop, the group would use empathy to understand the needs and pain points of app users, generate ideas for improving the app, and thereafter create prototypes to test with users. Through iteration and feedback from all users, the group would refine and improve the app until it met the needs of users and achieved the company's goals.

2.3.6 Sustainability-Focused Redesign

Sustainability-focused redesign aims to make a design more environmentally friendly and sustainable. It involves considering the lifecycle of the invention, from sourcing materials to manufacturing, usage, and disposal, and finding ways to minimize its environmental impact. This type of redesign often involves incorporating eco-friendly materials, reducing waste, and promoting energy efficiency.

It is important in the redesign rule because it addresses the urgent need to reduce the environmental impact of products and services. As the world's population grows and consumption increases, companies must prioritize sustainability in their design processes. By using design-thinking to create more sustainable products, companies can reduce waste, conserve resources, and minimize their carbon footprint. The sustainability-focused redesign also helps companies stay competitive by meeting the changing expectations of consumers, who are increasingly concerned about the environmental impact of their purchases. Finally, sustainability-focused redesign can lead to cost savings for companies by reducing waste and improving efficiency in the supply chain. Overall, sustainability-focused redesign is an essential element of responsible and forward-thinking design.

2.4 Tangibility Rule

According to this rule, tangible prototypes must be created to communicate their ideas effectively. Actual prototypes help designers understand which ideas work and which don't. This testing stage helps to create a seamless design process.

The tangibility rule in design-thinking refers to the principle of making ideas and concepts tangible and visible to facilitate communication, collaboration, and understanding among team members and stakeholders. The rule emphasizes the importance of creating physical or visual representations of ideas, such as sketches, prototypes, or mock-ups, to make them more concrete and easier to grasp.

By making ideas tangible, design thinkers can effectively communicate their vision, gather feedback, and iterate on their designs. Tangible representations also enable stakeholders to provide more specific and actionable feedback, as they can see and interact with the design in a more realistic way.

The tangibility rule also encourages designers to engage in hands-on experimentation and prototyping. By creating physical or digital prototypes, the ideas can be tested and validated, potential issues or challenges are uncovered, and their designs are refined based on real-world interactions and user feedback. There are several types of tangibility rules in design-thinking, including:

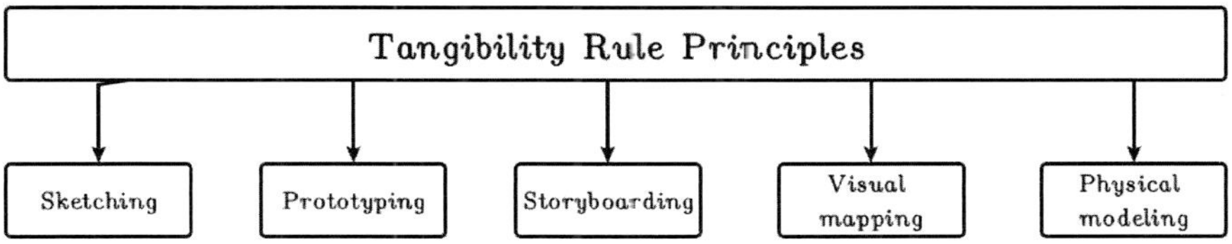

Figure 2.5: Tangibility Rule

2.4.1 Sketching

This involves creating quick and rough sketches or drawings to visualize and communicate ideas. Sketching allows designers to quickly iterate and explore different concepts and solutions.

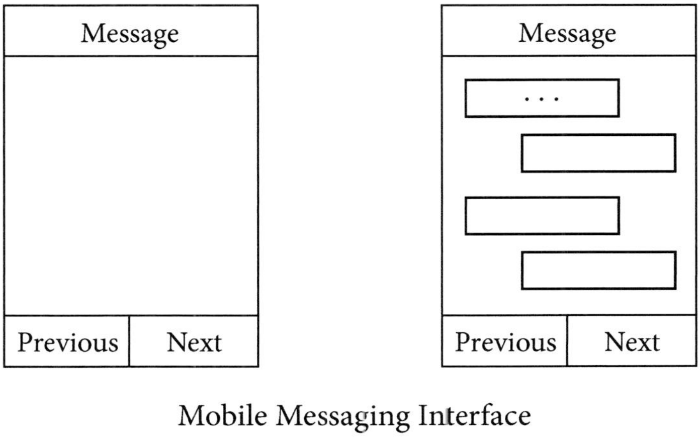

Figure 2.6: Mobile Messaging Interface Sketch

Sketching is important to the tangibility rule of design-thinking because it allows designers to visually represent their ideas and concepts. By sketching, different possibilities can be explored quickly, designs improved, and thoughts communicated to others.

Sketching helps make ideas more tangible and concrete, as it transforms abstract concepts into visual representations. This makes it easier for designers to understand and evaluate their ideas, identify potential issues or improvements, and make necessary adjustments.

Additionally, sketching promotes collaboration and communication within a design team or with stakeholders. It enables designers to share their ideas and receive feedback early in the design process, which helps in refining and enhancing the final design solution.

Overall, sketching plays a crucial role in the tangibility rule of design-thinking by providing a visual language that helps designers bring their ideas to life, evaluate their concepts, and effectively communicate with others involved in the design process.

2.4.2 Prototyping

This involves creating physical or digital prototypes of a design idea. Prototypes can range from low-fidelity mock-ups to high-fidelity representations that simulate the final product or experience. Prototyping helps designers test and gather feedback on their ideas, identify potential issues, and make improvements.

Prototyping is important to the tangibility rule of design-thinking because it allows designers to create physical or interactive representations of their ideas and concepts. By prototyping, designers can test and validate their designs, gather feedback from users or stakeholders, and make informed decisions about the final solution.

Prototyping helps make ideas tangible and concrete by providing a hands-on experience of the design. It allows designers to see how their ideas work in practice, identify any potential issues or challenges, and make necessary adjustments before investing significant time and resources into the final implementation.

Moreover, prototyping promotes collaboration and communication within a design team or with stakeholders. It enables designers to share their prototypes and gather feedback early in the design process, which helps in refining and improving the design solution based on real user insights.

Prototyping also helps reduce the risks and uncertainties associated with the design. By creating prototypes, designers can test different variations or alternatives, explore different functionalities or interactions, and evaluate the feasibility and viability of their ideas.

Overall, prototyping plays a crucial role in the tangibility rule of design-thinking by allowing designers to create physical or interactive representations of their ideas, test and validate their designs, gather feedback, and make informed decisions for the final solution. It helps in reducing risks, enhancing collaboration, and ensuring that the design meets the needs and expectations of the users.

Sketches and prototypes are both important tools in the design-thinking process, but they serve different purposes, as shown in Table 2.1

Table 2.1: Sketches vs Prototypes

Sketches	Prototypes
Sketches are typically quick, rough drawings that are used to explore and communicate ideas.	Prototypes are more detailed and refined representations of a design concept.
They are often created early in the design process before any detailed planning or prototyping has been done.	They are created later in the design process after sketches and other ideation activities have been completed.
Sketches are useful for exploring and communicating ideas.	Prototypes are essential for testing and refining
Sketches can be used to brainstorm new ideas, refine existing concepts, and communicate design concepts to stakeholders.	Prototypes can take many forms, from physical models to digital simulations, and they are used to test and refine the design concept

2.4.3 Storyboarding

This involves creating a sequence of visual illustrations or images to depict the user's journey or experience with a product or service. Storyboarding helps designers understand the user's perspective, identify pain points, and design solutions that address specific needs and goals.

Storyboarding is important in the tangibility rule of design-thinking because it helps designers visualize and communicate their ideas in a sequential and narrative format. By creating a series of sketches or illustrations, designers can tell a story that represents the user's journey or experience with the design solution (Mayfield, D, 2022).

Storyboarding allows designers to break down complex concepts or interactions into simple visual representations. It helps in structuring the flow of the design and identifying key moments or interactions that need to be considered. By visually mapping out the user's journey, designers can more comprehensively understand context and identify potential pain points or opportunities for improvement. An example of a storyboard for a food delivery app is shown in Figure 2.7.

Moreover, storyboarding helps in gathering feedback and aligning stakeholders' expectations. By presenting a storyboard, design visions can be effectively communicated engaging stakeholders in the design process. It

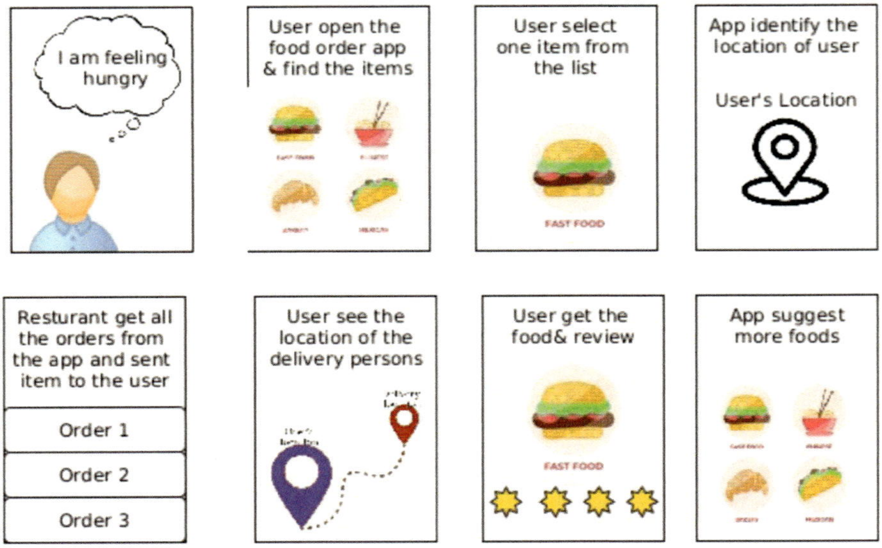

Figure 2.7: Example Storyboard for Food Delivery App

allows for early collaboration and discussion, enabling designers to gather valuable insights and make necessary adjustments before moving forward with prototyping.

Storyboarding also helps in evaluating the overall narrative and coherence of the design solution. By visualizing the user's journey, any gaps or inconsistencies can be identified in the flow and necessary revisions made. It allows for iterative refinement and ensures that the design solution provides a seamless and engaging experience for users.

Overall, storyboarding plays a crucial role in the tangibility rule of design-thinking by helping designers visualize and communicate their ideas, structure the flow of the design, gather feedback, and ensure a coherent and engaging user experience.

2.4.4 Visual Mapping

This involves creating visual representations, such as diagrams, flowcharts, or mind maps, to organize and communicate complex information or concepts. An example of a mind map for online shopping is shown in Figure 2.8. Visual mapping helps designers and stakeholders understand the connections and relationships between different elements of a design and identify potential areas for improvement or innovation (Interaction Design Foundation - IxDF, 2016).

Visual mapping is important in the tangibility rule of design-thinking because it helps designers create a tangible representation of ideas and concepts. By

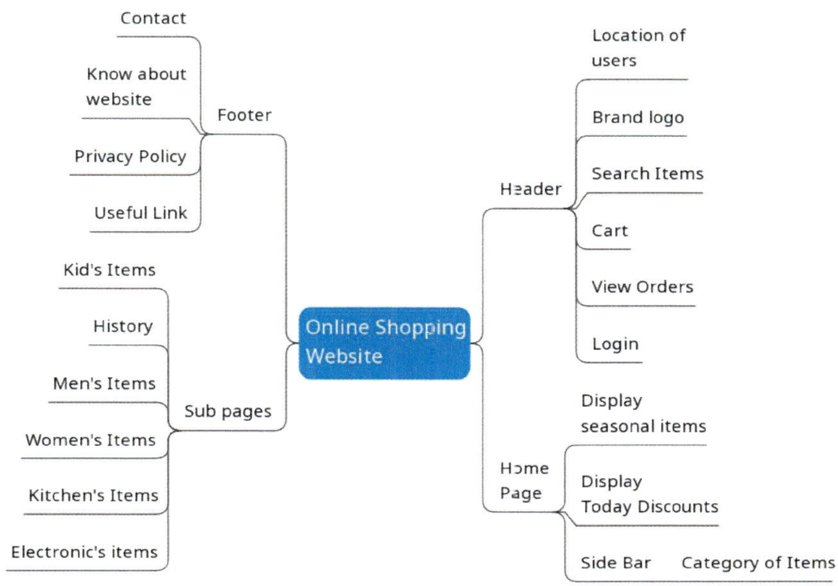

Figure 2.8: Mind-Map for Online Shopping

visually mapping out the design solution, their ideas can be made more concrete and easier to understand for both the designers and others.

Visual mapping allows designers to organize and structure their thoughts in a visual format. It helps in identifying the relationships between different elements of the design and how they fit together overall. By creating visual maps, designers can see the big picture and understand the overall structure and flow of the design.

Moreover, visual mapping aids in communication and collaboration. By creating visual representations, their ideas are communicated to stakeholders, team members, and clients. It provides a common language that everyone can understand and helps in aligning expectations and gaining buy-in from all parties involved.

Visual mapping also facilitates creativity and ideation. By visually representing ideas and concepts, different possibilities and variations can be explored. It allows for brainstorming and experimentation, enabling designers to generate new ideas and solutions.

Additionally, visual mapping helps in problem solving and decision making. By visually mapping out the design solution, potential issues or challenges can be identified and appropriate solutions developed. It allows for a systematic approach to problem solving and helps in making informed decisions based on visual analysis.

Overall, visual mapping is important in the tangibility rule of design-thinking because it helps designers create a tangible representation of their ideas, organize their thoughts, communicate effectively, facilitate creativity, and aid in problem solving and decision making.

2.4.5 Physical Modeling

This involves creating physical models or mock-ups of a design idea using materials like clay, foam, or 3D printing. Physical modeling explores the form, function, and ergonomics of a design and gathers feedback on its usability and aesthetics.

Physical modeling is important in the tangibility rule of design-thinking because it allows the creation of physical representations of ideas and concepts. By physically modeling the design solution, ideas can be made more tangible and easier to understand for both the designers and others (DesTechWiki., 2023).

Physical modeling provides a hands-on approach to design. It allows designers to manipulate and interact with physical materials, giving them a more comprehensive understanding of the form, function, and usability of the design. It tests and iterates ideas in a physical space, allowing for a more realistic evaluation of the design's feasibility and effectiveness.

Moreover, physical modeling aids in communication and collaboration. By creating physical prototypes, ideas can be effectively communicated to stakeholders, team members, and clients. It provides a tangible representation that everyone can see and touch, helping to align expectations and gaining buy-in from all parties involved.

Physical modeling also facilitates creativity and ideation. By physically manipulating materials and exploring different possibilities, new ideas and solutions can be generated. It allows for hands-on experimentation and encourages designers to think outside the box.

Additionally, physical modeling helps in problem solving and decision making. By physically prototyping the design solution, potential issues or challenges can be identified, and appropriate solutions can be developed. It allows for a more realistic evaluation of the design's functionality and usability, helping to make informed decisions based on physical analysis.

By employing these tangibility rules, designers can make their ideas more tangible and accessible, fostering more comprehensive communication, collaboration, and understanding among team members and stakeholders. Overall, the tangibility rule in design-thinking promotes a more collaborative and iterative approach to design, where ideas are made visible and tangible to foster more effective communication, understanding, and innovation.

2.5 Conclusion

Principles of design-thinking provide a framework for designers to navigate the complexities and uncertainties of the design process, helping them make informed decisions, stay focused on user needs, and create meaningful and impactful solutions.

References

Abell, A. and DeVore, K. 2017. Embracing ambiguity: a framework for promoting iterative design thinking approaches in engineering and design curricula. *In*: 2017 Asee Annual Conference and Exposition.

Dam, R.F and Siang, T.Y . 2022. Stakeholder mapping: the complete guide to stakeholder maps. https://www.interaction-design.org/literature/article/map-the-stakeholders. (Accessed: June 15, 2023).

Dunne, D. and Martin, R. 2006. Design thinking and how it will change management education: an interview and discussion. Academy of Management Learning and Education. 5(4): 512–523.

Interaction Design Foundation- IxDF. 2016. What is visual mapping?. interaction design foundation - ixdf. https://www.interaction-design.org/literature/topics/visual-mapping. (Accessed: October 06, 2022).

Mayfield, D. 2022. Guide to storyboards for design thinking. https://devsquad.com/blog/storyboards-design-thinking. (Accessed: September 18, 2023).

Meinel, C. and Leifer, L. 2011. Design thinking research. *In*: Design Thinking Research: Studying Co-creation in Practice. 1–11. Springer.

Tuusa, S. 2018. Re-designing the aesthetic of the future. https://medium.com/the-morrow/the-iphone-7a3cf5da76cb. (Accessed: July, 01, 2023).

DesTechWiki. 2023. 3.3 physical modelling. https://www.ruthtrumpold.id.au/destech/?page id=57. (Accessed: February 23, 2023).

Chapter 3

Phases of Design-Thinking

Design-thinking is a non-linear, iterative process with three to seven phases, depending on the challenge. This means that instead of adhering to a strict step-by-step procedure, it alternates between the various stages as new information and insights are obtained. This chapter focuses on the five-stage design-thinking model proposed by the Hasso Plattner Institute of Design at Stanford (commonly known as the d.school). First step involves identifying the problem and generating ideas for potential solutions through developing empathy for users' needs and experiences. Subsequently, user feedback, prototyping, and testing are used to refine and improve the solutions. This process is repeated until a final solution that addresses user needs and resolves the issues is created. Flexible approaches like design-thinking promote experimentation and learning, which can result in creative and useful solutions.

This chapter discusses the following phases of design-thinking:

- Empathize
- Define
- Ideate
- Prototype
- Test

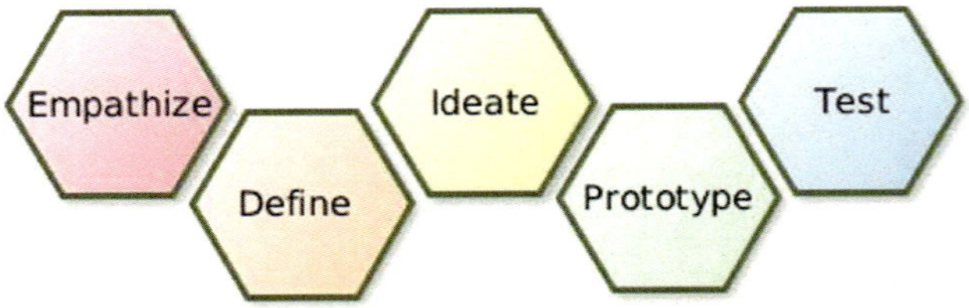

Figure 3.1: Five Phases of Design-Thinking

3.1 Empathize Research

Empathy is the first step in design-thinking as it allows designers to understand and experience the feelings of others. Through empathy, designers can put themselves in other people's shoes and connect with how they might be feeling about a given problem, circumstance, or situation. (Altman et al., 2018; McKenna, 2004) mentioned four primary methods of empathetic research.

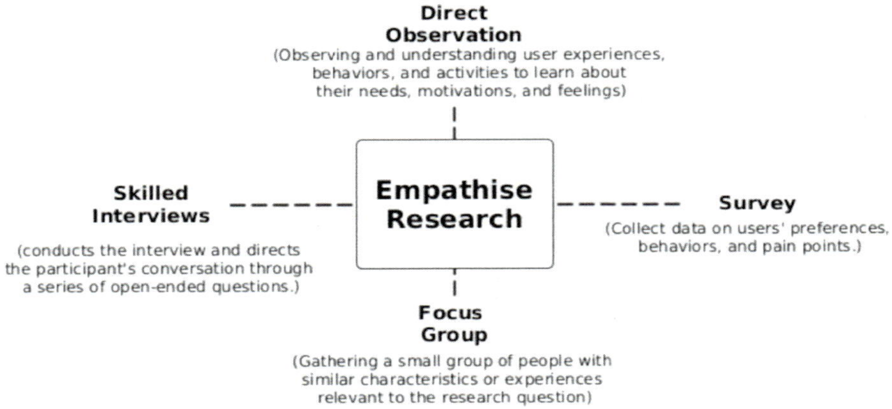

Figure 3.2: Types of Empathize Research

3.1.1 Direct Observation

Designers have the chance to empathize with users' experiences, comprehend their context, identify hidden needs, and hear their open and unfiltered feedback when they observe users in their natural environment. The act of intently seeing and comprehending another person's behaviors, activities, and experiences to obtain awareness of their needs, motives, and emotions is referred to as observation in the field of empathy research. To better comprehend the users' or customers' viewpoints and difficulties, one must immerse themselves in their environment and context (Author, P, 2019).

Direct observation of people in their natural environments, such as their homes, workplaces, or public locations, is frequently used in empathy research.

This gives designers the chance to see users' actual interactions with products, services, or locations and spot any pain points or unmet requirements.

In empathy research, observation goes beyond what people say they need or want. It aims to uncover the deeper motives, behaviors, and emotions driving their actions. Designers can learn more about consumers' experiences and find insights that might not be accessible through more conventional research techniques like interviews or surveys.

Being aware of prejudices and presumptions is also a necessary component of observation in empathy research. Designers must go into the observing process with an open mind and refrain from jumping to conclusions. They must be considerate of cultural variations, personal preferences, and the environment in which behaviors take place.

Finally, by carefully observing their surroundings, designers can gather important information that helps them build solutions that are more meaningful and effective. The effectiveness of the design-thinking process can be improved through insights since they can spark new ideas, point out areas for development, and pose theoretical conundrums.

3.1.2 Survey

A survey is a method of collecting data from a group of people by asking them a set of questions. In the context of design-thinking, surveys can be used to gather information about users' preferences, behaviors, and pain points.

To conduct a survey to empathize with research, designers may start by defining the research questions they want to answer. They can then create a survey questionnaire that includes open-ended and closed-ended questions. Open-ended questions allow participants to provide detailed responses, while closed-ended questions provide predefined response options for participants to choose from.

Once the survey is created, designers can distribute it to their target audience through various channels, such as email, social media, or online platforms. The collected data can then be analyzed to identify patterns and insights that inform the design process.

It is important to note that surveys are just one method of conducting empathizing research and should be used in conjunction with other methods such as skill interviews, direct observations, and focus groups to gain a holistic understanding of user needs and experiences.

3.1.3 Focus Groups

Focus groups are another technique used in empathy research to learn more about the desires, drives, and feelings of users and clients. A focus group often includes gathering a small number of people with comparable characteristics or experiences that are pertinent to the research issue.

An instructor leads a structured discussion in a focus group setting, inviting participants to express their ideas, opinions, and experiences regarding the subject at hand. For conversation starters and to encourage people to share their opinions, the facilitator may use open-ended questions or offer prompts.

By drawing on the collective knowledge and experiences of the members, focus groups are intended to produce rich qualitative data. It enables researchers to see and comprehend how people interact with one another, react to various stimuli, and shape each other's perspectives.

Focus groups offer participants the chance to think back on their experiences, tell stories, and talk about their feelings in a group context, which makes them particularly helpful in studies on empathy. Through group interviews or surveys, it is perhaps difficult to identify shared patterns, shared difficulties, and underlying motivations. Focus groups allow researchers to collect insights as well as non-verbal clues like body language and facial expressions, which can offer important context and improve comprehension of participants' emotions and behaviors.

It is crucial to remember that focus groups have limitations. Individual replies can be influenced by the dynamics of the group, and some individuals may experience pressure to hold back their genuine beliefs or conform to prevailing viewpoints. Furthermore, because of the small sample size, it is possible that the results do not accurately reflect the greater population. Despite these drawbacks, focus groups can be a useful tool for research on empathy when combined with other techniques. They give participants a forum to express their ideas and participate in the design process, which ultimately results in more empathetic and user-centered solutions.

3.1.4 Skilled Interviewing

Another technique used in empathy research to learn about desires, drives, and feelings of users or clients is skilled interviewing. Skilled interviewing, as opposed to focus groups, entails speaking with people individually who have relevant experiences or traits connected to the research topic.

In a skilled interview, the researcher conducts the interview and directs the participant's conversation. The interviewer encourages the participant to elaborate on their thoughts, opinions, and experiences by asking a series of open-ended questions or using other prompts. Interviewers with experience are taught to actively listen, elicit deeper insights, and foster a safe space for participants to express themselves.

The goal of a skillful interview is to delve deeply into a person's experiences and emotions so that researchers may fully comprehend their viewpoint. Researchers can use this technique to delve into the specifics of a person's thoughts and feelings, gaining novel insights that might not be accessible using other study methods.

Given the opportunity for participants to share their tales and experiences in a more private and intimate context, skilled interviewing can be particularly useful in studies examining empathy. A greater comprehension of a person's wants and desires results from giving people a secure environment in which to think about their feelings, motives, and difficulties.

Additionally, effective interviewing enables researchers to build a rapport with participants, foster trust, and persuade them to disclose sensitive or private information. As a result, the participant may respond more sincerely and openly, offering insightful details about their genuine emotions and experiences.

However, just like focus groups, skilled interviewing is not without its limitations. Because of the limited sample size, the results might not be representative of a larger population. Additionally, elements like the interviewer's own prejudices or the social desirability bias can have an impact on a person's responses.

Skillful interviewing is sometimes combined with other research techniques, such as focus groups or observation, to overcome limitations. Researchers can gain a more thorough and nuanced understanding of users' or customers' requirements, motives, and emotions by combining several methodologies, which will ultimately results in more sympathetic and user-centered solutions.

The D. School at Stanford has developed the following set of guidelines for empathy interviews (Zaldarriaga, A., 2016):

- Start the interview by asking *"why"*. Even if the interviewers believe they know the answer, they should still ask people why they do or say things. Interviewers will occasionally be surprised by the answers. A conversation should begin with a single question and last as long as necessary.
- Never use *"usually"* when asking a question. Instead, inquire about a specific instance or occurrence, like *"Tell me about the last time."*
- Encourage people to share stories. Whether or not the stories are true, they show how people perceive the world. Ask questions that encourage people to share their stories.
- Look for inconsistencies. Sometimes what people say and what they do are different. These inconsistencies often hide interesting insights.
- Pay attention to nonverbal cues. Be aware of body language and emotions.
- Maintain silence whenever needed. When there is a pause during an interview, interviewers frequently feel compelled to ask another question. If the interviewer allows for silence, a person can reflect on what they've just said, potentially revealing something deeper.

- Suggesting answers to questions is not permitted. Even if people pause before responding, avoid attempting to suggest an answer. This can unintentionally cause people to say things consistent with their beliefs.
- Maintain neutrality when asking questions. For example, "What do you think about buying gifts for your spouse?" is preferable to "Don't you think shopping is great?" because the former encourages open responses without leading the person to a specific conclusion.
- Avoid asking binary questions. Binary questions can be answered in a single word, and the interviewers want to facilitate a conversation based on stories.
- Make sure to prepare for capture. Always interview in pairs. If this is not possible, interviewers may benefit greatly from using a voice recorder. It is impossible to properly engage a user and take detailed notes at the same time.

3.1.5 Direct Observation vs Surveys vs Focus Groups vs Skill Interviews

Table 3.1 clarifies the purposes of each method, making it easier to choose the right one for specific research or evaluation needs.

3.2 Define

The defining step in design-thinking comes after the empathize phase in the design process. It is centered on developing a thorough understanding of the issue or challenge at hand and defining it in a way that directs the remaining design steps. The problem or challenge is defined during the define phase by designers and researchers using a variety of tools and methods. The data and insights obtained throughout the empathize phase must be combined to create problem statements that can be addressed effectively. This phase aims to include Reframing the problem and creating a problem statement.

Reframing involves reframing the initial problem or challenge statement based on insights and data collected during empathy phase. It may involve identifying the underlying issues and root causes that need to be addressed. Creating a problem statement is another aspect of this phase. A problem statement is a concise and clear description of the problem or challenge that needs to be solved. It should be framed in a way that focuses on user needs and motivations. The problem statement provides a guiding principle for the rest of the design process.

Table 3.1: Direct Observation vs Surveys vs Focus Groups vs Skill Interviews

Direct Observation	Surveys	Focus Groups	Skill Interviews
Direct observation is the process of observing people or events in their natural settings without interference.	Surveys involve collecting data through questionnaires or interviews.	Focus groups involve bringing together a group of people to discuss a specific topic or issue.	Skill interviews involve assessing an individual's skills and abilities through a structured interview.
Direct observation is valuable for collecting data on behaviors, interactions, and patterns.	Surveys can be conducted in person, over the phone, or online. Surveys are useful for gathering data on attitudes, opinions, and behaviors.	The group is led by a moderator who asks questions and facilitates discussion. Focus groups help gather data on attitudes, opinions, and perceptions.	Skill interviews are useful for gathering data on job-related skills and abilities.
Direct observation can be structured involving setting up a specific protocol for observing and recording data, or it can be unstructured which allows for more flexibility in data collection.	Surveys can be open-ended, where questions allow for more detailed responses, or it can be closed-ended, where questions provide more structured responses.	Focus groups allow for in-depth exploration of a topic and can provide insights into how people think and feel about a particular issue.	Skill interviews can be used to assess an individual's knowledge, experience, and qualifications for a specific job or task.
Direct observation is useful when the researcher wants to see how people behave in real-life situations.	Surveys are useful when the researcher wants to gather information from a large number of people.	Focus groups are useful when the researcher wants to gather information from a specific group of people.	Skill interviews are useful when the researcher wants to assess an individual's skills and abilities.

3.2.1 Developing User Personas

User personas are fictional representations of different types of users or customers (Pesot, J. and Plantenberg, S., 2023). They are created based on research and data collected during the empathy phase. User personas are used to understand the various needs, goals, and characteristics of the target audience. Personas are important tools for defining problem. They are discussed in more details in the following chapter. Once the personas are created, then an empathy map will be created to articulate what designers know about a particular type of user. For example, if the persona is a busy working mother, the empathy map may include sections for her thoughts about balancing work and family responsibilities, her feelings of stress and guilt, her actions of juggling multiple tasks, and her environment of a busy household. By using personas to inform inquiry, a deeper understanding of the user's experience can be gained, and solutions created that better meet their needs.

3.2.2 Journey Mapping

Journey mapping is a visual representation of the customer's journey through a product or service. It helps to identify the pain points and challenges that the customer faces during the journey. The journey mapping process involves defining the problem by understanding the customer's needs, wants, and expectations. For instance, the steps depicted in Figure 3.3 might be included in a customer journey map for a mobile banking app. This tool is explained broadly in the next chapter.

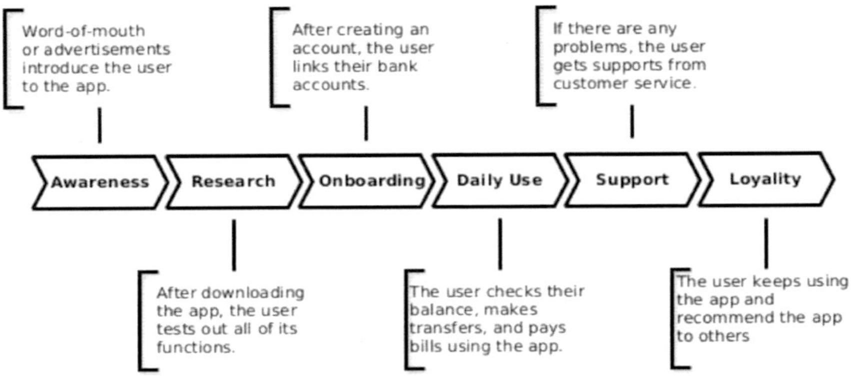

Figure 3.3: Customer Journey Map for a Mobile Banking App

3.2.3 Creating a Point Of View (POV) statement

The point of view (POV) statement is a concise and focused statement that captures the customer's perspective and pain points at a specific touchpoint in their journey. For instance, as Figure 3.3 illustrates, some users may find the onboarding process confusing, which could cause them to become frustrated and stop using the app. Designers can develop solutions that improve the onboarding process's intuitiveness and usability by recognizing these pain points. The statement is written from the customer's point of view and includes their thoughts, feelings, and needs. The POV statement helps to clarify the problem and provides a clear direction for developing solutions. It is an essential component of the journey mapping process as it helps to align the team's understanding of the customer's experience and prioritize areas for improvement.

The define phase is crucial in design-thinking as it sets the direction and scope for the rest of the design process. It ensures that designers have a clear understanding of the problem or challenge they are trying to solve and helps them stay focused on the user's needs and motivations.

3.3 Ideate

During the ideate phase, a range of concepts and potential solutions can be generated to address the given problem. The design process moves on to the third stage of design-thinking, known as *Ideate*, following the define phase. The main goal is to generate a wide range of creative and innovative ideas to address a particular problem or challenge. To produce as many ideas as possible during the ideation phase, several kinds of brainstorming sessions and other creative exercises are conducted. The goal of brainstorming is to encourage divergent thinking and explore different perspectives and options. The following actions are commonly included in the Ideate phase:

3.3.1 Brainstorming

Design-thinking uses brainstorming as a technique to produce innovative concepts and solutions to problems. It entails a group of people discussing their ideas and opinions in a transparent and accepting environment. Let us take the scenario where a design team is assigned to develop a new product for a fitness company. To come up with ideas for the product, the team decided to conduct brainstorming sessions. Team members are encouraged to share any ideas that come to mind during the brainstorming session, regardless of how unusual or impractical they may seem.

As an illustration of the brainstorm, consider a smartwatch that tracks a user's heart rate, steps taken, and calories burned in addition to offering personalized workout recommendations based on the user's fitness level and goals. The group can evaluate ideas to determine which ones are realistic and fit the project goals after brainstorming session. Once a successful product has been developed, the most promising ideas can be tested and prototyped.

3.3.2 Crazy 8s

The *crazy 8s* method can be used during the ideation stage. This involves folding a piece of paper into eight equal parts. Following that, each team member has eight minutes to generate eight different ideas, one for each section. This encourages creativity and innovation and allows for quick brainstorming sessions. Following the crazy 8s exercise, the group can evaluate and deliberate on each concept before deciding which ideas are most viable. This makes it easier to ensure that everyone on the team has an equal opportunity to contribute and that different ideas are considered.

3.3.3 Mind Mapping

Once the team has generated a list of ideas through brainstorming, they can use mind mapping to organize and expand upon them. Mind mapping is a visual technique that involves creating a diagram that connects different ideas and concepts. By using mind mapping, the team can explore different aspects of each idea and identify potential challenges and opportunities. This helps in refining ideas and creating more detailed plan for prototyping and testing. This tool is discussed broadly in Chapter 5.

3.3.4 SCAMPER

SCAMPER is a powerful ideation technique that can be used in the ideate phase after mind mapping. The acronym stands for Substitute, Combine, Adapt, Modify, Put to another use, Eliminate, and Reverse as shown in Figure 3.4. Each of these prompts can be used to generate new ideas based on existing concepts.

S	C	A	M	P	E	R
Substitute	Combine	Adapt	Modify	Put to another use	Eliminate	Reverse
This prompt involves substituting one element of an idea with another	This prompt involves combining two or more ideas to create a new solution	This prompt involves adapting an existing product or service for a new market or audience.	This prompt involves modifying an existing feature to better meet user needs	This prompt involves using an idea in a different context or industry	This prompt involves eliminating a feature that is not essential or adding unnecessary complexity	This prompt involves reversing the order of steps in a process.

Figure 3.4: Scamper

By using SCAMPER in the ideate phase, teams can challenge assumptions and generate new ideas based on existing concepts. This can help identify unique solutions that may not have been considered otherwise.

The Ideate phase is crucial in design-thinking as it allows for the exploration of a wide range of ideas and possibilities. It encourages creativity, collaboration, and innovation, which can lead to breakthrough solutions. The ideas generated during this phase will be further evaluated and refined in the next phase of the design process, the prototype phase.

3.4 Prototype

The prototype phase in design-thinking is the stage where physical or digital models of ideas are created to test and gather feedback. It involves building a representation of the proposed solution, which can range from low-fidelity sketches to high-fidelity interactive prototypes.

The main purpose of prototyping is to quickly and cheaply explore different design options and gather user feedback. By creating a tangible representation of the solution, it is possible to more comprehensively understand how it might work in the real world and identify any potential flaws or areas of improvements.

For example, a team could create a prototype smartwatch design, including the placement of buttons, the size and shape of the screen, and any other physical features. They could then create a digital prototype using software like Figma or Sketch, which would allow them to test different design options and simulate user interactions.

The prototype phase often follows an iterative approach including creating a prototype, testing it with users, gathering feedback, and then refining the design based on the insights gained. This process is repeated multiple times to learn from failures, make necessary adjustments, and continuously improve solutions.

Prototypes can take various forms, depending on the nature of the project. They can be physical models made from materials like paper, cardboard, or foam, or they can be digital mockups created using design software or prototyping tools. The choice of prototype type depends on the specific needs of the project and the level of fidelity required to effectively communicate and test the design.

The prototype phase is crucial in design-thinking because it allows designers to validate their assumptions, uncover potential issues early on, and gather valuable user feedback before investing significant time and resources into development. It helps designers refine their ideas, make informed design decisions, and ultimately create solutions that better meet user needs. Prototyping methods are generally divided into two separate categories: low-fidelity prototyping and high-fidelity prototyping.

3.4.1 Low-Fidelity Prototypes

These prototypes are quick and inexpensive to create and are often made using simple materials like paper, cardboard, or sticky notes. They are used to explore and communicate basic concepts and interactions. Low-fidelity prototypes in design-thinking are simple and basic representations of a product or service, created using inexpensive materials or digital tools. These prototypes are often quick and easy to create, allowing designers to explore and test different ideas and concepts early in the design process.

Low-fidelity prototypes are intentionally rough and incomplete, focusing on the core functionality or key features of the design. They may include sketches, paper mock-ups, wireframes, or basic digital mock-ups. These prototypes are not intended to look polished or realistic, but rather to communicate the basic structure and functionality of the design.

The purpose of low-fidelity prototypes is to gather feedback and insights from users and stakeholders at an early stage of the design process. By creating and testing these prototypes, designers can quickly iterate and refine their ideas based on user feedback without investing significant time or resources in developing a fully functional prototype. Examples of low-fidelity prototypes are:

- **Storyboarding:** entails creating a visual narrative of a user's interaction with a product or service. It is frequently used to show how a user might interact with a product or service over time, from discovery to final use.
- **Sketching:** refers to the process of creating rough, hand-drawn sketches or diagrams of initial design concepts for a product or service. Sketching is a low-fidelity method for quickly exploring different design ideas and visualizing how they might work in practice.
- **Card-Sorting:** is a prototype design-thinking technique that helps designers organize and categorize information in a way that makes sense to users. It entails creating a set of cards with various pieces of information, such as features, functions, or content, and asking users to group them based on their criteria.
- **Wizard of Oz:** is used in design-thinking to simulate a user experience even when the technology or product being tested is not yet functional. The name is derived from the classic story in which the wizard creates the illusion of power and control even though he is only a man behind a curtain.

Low-fidelity prototypes are particularly useful for exploring different design options, validating assumptions, and identifying potential usability issues or improvements. They provide a tangible representation of the design concept that can be easily modified or discarded as needed, allowing designers to make informed decisions and move forward in the design process.

3.4.2 High-Fidelity Prototypes

High-fidelity prototypes are detailed and fully functional representations of a product or service that closely resemble the final version. In design-thinking, high-fidelity prototypes are created in the later stages of the design process, after low-fidelity prototypes have been tested and refined. High-fidelity prototypes are typically created using advanced design tools and materials, such as computer-aided design (CAD) software, 3D printing, or other rapid prototyping techniques. They are designed to look and feel like the final product, with realistic textures, colors, and materials.

High-fidelity prototypes are used to test and refine the product or service before it is launched. They allow designers to identify any issues or problems with the product's functionality, usability, or aesthetics, and make any necessary changes before it goes into production. Overall, high-fidelity prototypes are an essential tool in the design-thinking process, as they allow designers to create and test realistic representations of their ideas and ensure that the final product meets the needs of users.

3.4.2.1 Low-Fidelity Prototypes vs High-Fidelity Prototypes

Table 3.2 highlights the key differences in detail, tools, purpose, and costs between the two types of prototypes.

Table 3.2: Low-Fidelity Prototype vs High-Fidelity Prototype

Aspect	Low-Fidelity Prototype	High-Fidelity Prototype
Level of Detail	Low-fidelity prototypes are rough, simple, and basic representations of a product or service.	High-fidelity prototypes are detailed and fully functional representations that closely resemble the final version.
Materials and Tool	Low-fidelity prototypes are often made using low-cost materials such as paper, cardboard, or foam, and can be created using basic tools like scissors and glue	High-fidelity prototypes are typically created using advanced design tools and materials such as computer-aided design (CAD) software, 3D printing, or other rapid prototyping techniques.
Purpose	Low-fidelity prototypes are used to quickly test and iterate on design ideas.	High-fidelity prototypes are used to test and refine the product or service before it is launched
Time and Cost	Low-fidelity prototypes can be created quickly and at low cost.	High-fidelity prototypes take longer to create and can be more expensive.

Prototyping allows designers to test their ideas and concepts in a low-risk environment, identify potential issues, and refine their design before moving on to the testing phase.

3.5 Test

The *Test phase* in design-thinking is the stage where designers evaluate their prototypes and gather feedback from users to assess the effectiveness and usability of their proposed solutions. The main objective of this phase is to validate the design assumptions, identify any issues or areas for improvement, and make informed decisions for further development.

User testing sessions are carried out during the test phase, where users are observed interacting with the prototypes. Gaining insight into user preferences and needs facilitates the identification of any usability problems or pain points as well as the comprehension of how users perceive and utilize the solution.

Numerous techniques, including surveys, observation, interviews, and usability testing, can be used during the testing process. Users may be questioned specifically about their experiences, their actions and reactions observed, and both quantitative and qualitative data gathered for analysis and design decision-making. Based on the feedback and insights gathered during testing, iteration, and refinement can be conducted. This iterative approach allows designers to continuously improve their designs, address any identified issues or concerns, and ensure that the final solution meets user needs and expectations.

The test phase is crucial in design-thinking because it provides valuable feedback and insights that help designers make informed decisions and improve their solutions. By involving users early in the process, expensive mistakes can be avoided, and solutions are more likely to be successful in the real world. Additionally, the test phase helps designers build empathy with users, understand their perspectives, and ensure that the final solution truly addresses their needs and desires.

3.5.1 The Goal of the Testing Phase

After testing is completed, the end product or service satisfies design-thinking's ultimate objective. Design-thinking ultimately aims to produce viable, feasible, and desirable solutions. The *Desirable-Feasible-Viable* (DFV) framework, which comprises these three criteria, represents the essential factors that designers need to take into account to guarantee the effectiveness and durability of their solutions. According to Kitch, B (2023), the DFV works in the following ways:

3.5.1.1 Desirable

The solution developed must be something that customers desire, not just something that they find appealing.

- **User-Centric:** end users' requirements, preferences, and experiences have to be at the core of any solution. The goal of designers is to provide useful, pleasurable, and emotionally compelling products and services.
- **Empathy:** a key component of design-thinking is user empathy. Creating solutions that appeal to users requires an understanding of their context, motivations, and challenges.

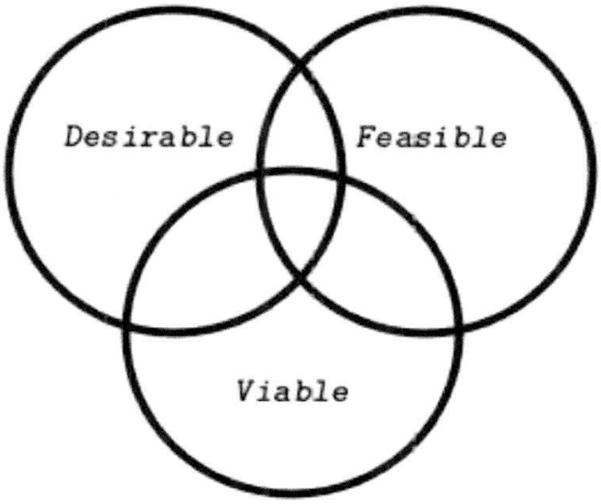

Figure 3.5: Desirable Feasible Viable

3.5.1.2 Feasible

Feasibility ensures that product concepts are only viable if the designers have access to all the resources required for development and up-to-date technology.

- **Technologically and Operationally Viable:** Technically and operationally viable solutions are required. This indicates that considering available technology, resources, and capabilities, the proposed concepts can be implemented realistically.
- **Realistic Implementation:** Feasibility takes into account the practical aspects of implementing a solution, accounting for resource availability, technological limitations, and any other relevant factors.

3.5.1.3 Viable

Designers must ensure that there exist an approprite market; a small audience interested in their concept cannot sustain a successful business:

- **Financial Viability**: economic sustainability is a feature of viable solutions. From a business standpoint, ideas must make sense, taking into account prospective revenue streams along with the expenses of development, production, and maintenance.
- **Scalability:** viable solutions can grow and change to satisfy shifting needs. They are capable of increasing in size and scope without losing their efficacy.

A balanced and comprehensive approach to problem-solving is ensured by the integration of these three factors. These elements function cohesively as follows:

- **Balancing Trade-Offs:** designers often need to make trade-offs between desirability, feasibility, and viability. For example, a highly desirable feature is perhaps technically challenging to implement, or a feasible solution may not align with the organization's financial goals. Designers must find the optimal balance among these factors.
- **Iterative Process**: achieving a desirable, feasible, and viable solution is an iterative process. Designers go through cycles of ideation, prototyping, testing, and refinement to converge on a solution that meets all three criteria.
- **Cross-Functional Collaboration:** successful implementation of the DFV framework often requires collaboration among cross-functional teams, including designers, engineers, business professionals, and other stakeholders. This interdisciplinary collaboration ensures that solutions are well-rounded and address various perspectives.

In summary, the end goal of design-thinking is to deliver solutions that not only meet user needs and preferences (desirable) but are also feasible to implement from a technical standpoint and viable in terms of economic sustainability. This comprehensive approach helps organizations create innovative and impactful solutions that with stand the test of time.

3.5.2 Tools for Testing

In the testing phase of design-thinking, designers use a variety of tools to gather feedback and insights from users. Some common tools used in this phase include:

- **User Testing:** this involves observing users as they interact with prototypes and asking them questions about their experience.
- **Analytics:** designers may use analytics tools to track user behavior and gather data on how users interact with their prototypes.
- **A/B Testing:** involves testing two different versions of a prototype to see which performs better with users.

Testing in design-thinking is the process of evaluating and gathering feedback on a product or service through various methods to validate and improve its design. It involves conducting experiments, observations, and assessments to understand user needs, preferences, and behaviors. Testing helps designers identify potential issues, refine their designs, and make data-driven decisions to create user-centered solutions. It is an iterative process that occurs throughout the design-thinking cycle to ensure that the final product or service meets user expectations and delivers a positive user experience.

Chapter 5 goes into great detail about theses testing tools. The main objective of the testing phase is to collect input and observations that will help enhance and improve the design solution.

3.6 Conclusion

This chapter has briefly discussed all phases of the design-thinking process, including empathize, define, ideate, prototype, and test. These phases are not necessarily linear and can be iterative, meaning that designers may cycle back and forth between different phases as they learn from testing and gather new insights. The design-thinking process is characterized by its user-centered approach and emphasis on iteration and refinement based on user feedback.

References

Kitch, B. 2023. Testing: a guide to the 5th stage of design thinking. https://www.mural.co/blog/design-thinking-testing. (Accessed: December 22, 2023)

Altman, M., Huang, T.T. and Breland, J.Y. 2018. Peer reviewed: design thinking in health care. Preventing Chronic Disease. 15.

Author, P. 2019. Design thinking: wmpathy and observation (pt 3). https://blogs.perficient.com/2019/01/16/design-thinking-empathy-observation-pt-3/. (Accessed: July 06, 2023).

McKenna, C.K. 2004. Chapter 9—listening to stakeholders: interviews, focus groups, surveys, and direct observation. *In*: J.T. Ziegenfuss and J.W. Sassani (eds). Portable Health Administration. 173–184. San Diego: Academic Press. Retrieved from https://www.sciencedirect.com/science/article/pii/B978012780590050050X doi: https://doi.org/10.1016/B978-012780590-0/50050-X

Pesot, J. and Plantenberg, S. 2023. Define personas —ibm garage practices. https://www.ibm.com/garage/method/practices/think/ practice personas/. (Accessed: October 09, 2023).

Zaldarriaga, A. 2016. Design thinking empathy: a guide to empathetic innovation. https://www.tlpnyc.com/blog/design-thinking-empathy.(Accessed: Accessed: December 29, 2023).

Chapter 4

Design-Thinking in Practice

This chapter will present case studies and real-world examples of how businesses and individuals have effectively used design-thinking techniques to address challenging issues and spur innovation. Empathy, cooperation, and iteration are prioritized so that businesses may drive innovation and develop products and experiences that connect with their target market. In the chapter, examples are offered that show how businesses have applied design-thinking to comprehend customer needs, generate original ideas, and develop solutions that significantly improve people's lives. Design-thinking has been used by many successful businesses to innovate and set themselves apart from rivals. Enginess (2023) provides examples that discuss the following topics:

- Airbnb
- Apple
- IDEO
- IBM
- Stanford d.school
- Ford

4.1 Airbnb

Airbnb used design-thinking to upend the established hotel business. This business recognized an opportunity to match those who have spare space with others who need lodging by empathizing with traveler needs and difficulties. The way people travel and locate lodging has been completely transformed through the Airbnb's platform, which was improved through iterative development and testing. Joe Gebbia, Nathan Blecharczyk, and Brian Chesky established Airbnb in 2008.

4.1.1 Background

Chesky went to San Francisco in 2007 to live with Gebbia, a designer and former classmate at the Rhode Island School of Design, after quitting his work as a designer on a famous TV show. During the annual Industrial Design Society of America Conference in October 2007, all the hotels in San Francisco were fully booked, making it impossible for conference attendees to obtain lodging.

The two roommates, who were having trouble paying the rent, decided to "make a few bucks" by taking advantage of the difficulty. With three air mattresses provided, they rented out space in their apartment. They added the promise of breakfast to make the deal more alluring. The website *"airbedandbreakfast.com"* was created by the two friends. To their amazement, the plan was successful, and six days later they received three guests—two men and a lady. Each night, the guests paid about $80 each. The venture was successful, which inspired young business people to expand upon it.

4.1.2 Turnaround with Design-Thinking

Airbnb was about to go out of business in 2009. The company barely made $200 a week in revenue. In a situation where survival was at risk, the founders started to analyze the format of their product advertisements. They were able to identify the issue after some consideration. They discovered that because the owners were utilizing camera phones, the photos of the houses that were displayed on the website were ugly. In addition, not all rooms in the house were displayed, which prevented consumers from booking rooms because they could not clearly understand what they were paying for. According to Gebbia, "It was not a surprise that people were not booking rooms because designers couldn't even really see what people were paying for" (Ellis, 2015).

4.1.3 Redesigning the Booking Process

Airbnb used design-thinking to improve the booking process on its platform. Researchers conducted interviews and observed users to identify pain points and areas for improvement (Cheng, Vivian, 2018). Through multiple user research projects and interviews, they arrived at some key insights:

- The user desired information as quickly as possible (for instance, regular homes rather than experiences, *Home Plus*, or other recommendations).

- The *Save* or *Location* function was not used by users in decision-making(many chose to disregard it).
- Users frequently delayed booking process and began comprising other options, as Users were unsure how to effectively compare the different options, and led them to rely on other comparison methods.

As a result, Airbnb introduced features like a map view, personalized recommendations, and a wish list to make it easier for users to find and book accommodations. Below are some features of the booking system in Airbnb.

- **Search:** guests can search using a variety of filters, including area, dates, price range, home type, and facilities.
- **Booking Request:** after finding a listing that appeals to them, guests can contact the host with a booking request. The request must be accepted or rejected by the host within 24 hours.
- **Payment:** through Airbnb's secure payment system, guests can pay for their reservations using a variety of options, including credit cards, PayPal, and Apple Pay.
- **Confirmation**: guests get an email with information about their reservation as soon as the host approves their booking request and the payment is finalized.
- **Communication:** before and throughout their stay, guests can get in touch with hosts using Airbnb's messaging service.
- **Review**: both guests and hosts can submit reviews for one another following their stay, which promotes mutual respect and enhances the Airbnb community as a whole.

4.1.4 Enhancing Trust and Safety

The Airbnb experience is crucially dependent on trust and safety. To address this, Airbnb used design-thinking to develop functions that would improve host-guest trust. As a result of their investigation into consumer concerns, features including verified profiles, safe payments, and a review system were created. These architectural adjustments sought to increase confidence and give assurance to both hosts and guests (Walsh et al., 2020). According to Joe Gebbia's 2016 TED talk, Airbnb is aware that trust and safety are essential components of its platform. The *"Trust & Safety"* division at AirBnB handles issues related to travel, hosting, community standards, and personal safety. Strong reputational processes on the platform can combat bias and increase trust, according to research done in collaboration with Stanford University. It uses three reputational mechanisms to assist users in overcoming their fear of interacting with strangers:

- **Profile:** to use the Airbnb site, both hosts and guests must first create a profile. Full name, phone number, payment details, and email address are just a few of the fields found in a basic profile. Also required are pictures of the accommodation from the hosts.
- **Secure Messaging:** for communication between the guest and the host, the site offers a secure messaging feature. The two parties may utilize it for coordination and to exchange further information or requests.
- **Reviews:** after a reservation, guests and hosts can rate each other in reviews, which is undoubtedly the most effective reputational tool on AirBnB. The Stanford study discovered that text reviews and the rating system are effective trust-maintenance tools.

To strengthen its trust ecosystem, AirBnB launched a superhost programme. Through this programme, exceptional hosts can earn the title of *"superhost"* if they meet the following requirements: an average rating of 4.8 or higher out of 5, completion of at least 10 trips or 100 nights over the last three completed stays, a cancellation rate of less than 1%, and a response rate of more than 90%. Superhosts gain advantages by being highlighted on the platform, drawing in more hosts, and earning more rewards from the platform. On the AirBnB platform, there are about 400,000 superhosts, or about 10% of all hosts. Furthermore, Airbnb offers the following features to increase the platform's credibility and security (FasterCapital, 2024):

- **Account Protection:** AirBnB uses multi-factor authentication on its platform to protect user accounts whenever a login attempt is made from a different device or location. Additionally, it notifies users anytime there is a transaction or account update.
- **Prevention of Fraud:** AirBnB offers multiple layers of defense against scammers. To do this, fraudulent postings are detected using a machine learning application, contact information is withheld until a reservation is confirmed, and payments are only released after check-in. Therefore, users are safe from scammers as long as they remain on the platform and communicate there.
- **Secure Payments:** AirBnB only accepts payments through its platform, discouraging customers from using wire transfers or cash to make payments. This aids in guaranteeing the transactions' security and traceability.
- **Risk Scoring:** machine learning and predictive analytics are used by AirBnB to assign a risk score to each reservation. Numerous flags from previous transactions are used to calculate the scores.
- **Watchlists and Background Checks:** AirBnB regularly verifies that its hosts and visitors are not on any sanctions, regulatory, or terrorist watchlists. For its US clients, it also runs its background checks.

- **Home Preparedness:** along with regional authorities, AirBnB offers home safety seminars with hosts. Guests are expected to receive important local information from hosts. If requested, the company also offers complimentary smoke and/or carbon monoxide alarms to the hosts. They are very clear in their host policy about the use of concealed cameras: "Spying on others is not appropriate; cameras are not allowed in the listing unless they have been previously disclosed and visible, and they are never permitted in private spaces (such as bathrooms or sleeping areas)."

4.1.5 Improving the Host Experience

Airbnb recognized the importance of providing a seamless experience for hosts as well. They used design-thinking to identify pain points in the host journey, such as difficulties in managing bookings and communication with guests. Through user research and prototyping, Airbnb introduced features like a hosted dashboard, messaging tools, and automated check-in instructions to simplify the hosting process and improve overall satisfaction for hosts.

- **Host Protection Insurance:** in the extremely unlikely event that the home or possessions are harmed by a guest while they are staying at their Airbnb listing, host damage protection, a component of *AirCover for Hosts*, offers $3 million in coverage.
- **Host Liability Insurance:** as part of *AirCover for Hosts*, host liability insurance offers $1 million in coverage in the unlikely event that hosts are held legally liable for a guest's injury or the damage or theft of their goods while they are staying at the accomodation.
- **Host Resources:** Airbnb provides hosts with a variety of resources, including a host community forum, educational resources, and support from customer service representatives.
- **Smart Pricing:** Airbnb's *Smart Pricing* tool helps hosts set competitive prices for their listings based on factors such as demand, seasonality, and local events.
- **Superhost Program**: Airbnb's Superhost program recognizes and rewards hosts who consistently provide exceptional hospitality to their guests. *Superhosts* receive benefits such as increased visibility in search results and exclusive invitations to events and workshops.

4.1.6 Designing for Inclusivity

Airbnb also applied design-thinking principles to address inclusivity and accessibility challenges. They conducted research to understand the needs of diverse user groups, including people with disabilities. Based on these insights,

Airbnb made design changes such as adding accessibility filters, providing detailed accessibility information for listings, and partnering with organizations that focus on accessible travel. These efforts aimed to make travel more inclusive and accessible for all users.

- **Accessibility Filters:** Airbnb offers accessibility filters that allow guests to search for listings that meet specific accessibility needs, such as wheelchair accessibility or step-free access.
- **Inclusive Design Guidelines:** Airbnb has developed inclusive design guidelines that help hosts create listings that are welcoming and accessible to all guests, regardless of their abilities or backgrounds.
- **Translation Services:** Airbnb offers translation services for hosts and guests who speak different languages, making it easier for people from different cultures and backgrounds to communicate and connect.
- **Non-Discrimination Policy:** Airbnb has a strict non-discrimination policy that prohibits hosts from discriminating against guests based on their race, ethnicity, gender identity, sexual orientation, or any other protected characteristic.
- **Inclusive Experiences:** Airbnb offers a range of inclusive experiences that celebrate diverse cultures and communities, including food tours, art classes, and cultural workshops.
- **Community Commitment:** Airbnb is committed to creating a more inclusive and welcoming community, and works to promote diversity and inclusion through partnerships with organizations like the NAACP and the National Urban League.

Overall, these case studies demonstrate how Airbnb utilized design-thinking to identify user needs, develop innovative solutions, and enhance the overall user experience on its platform.

4.2 Apple

Apple is known for its design-thinking approach to creating products that are not only aesthetically pleasing but also intuitive and user-friendly. They extensively prioritize user experience and research to understand their target audience's needs and pain points (Elmansy, R., 2016). This approach has allowed them to create groundbreaking products like the iPhone and iPad, revolutionizing the tech industry. Steve Jobs put design-thinking into practice by setting certain priorities, according to Chaturvedi, N. (2020).

- The needs of people take priority over the needs of businesses.
- Designs for products that fascinate people.

- Apple has become a status symbol for many people, signifying luxury and wealth.
- Focus on design over engineering
- Product simplicity and minimalism are preferred over complexity.

Apple was not always what it is now; from 1985 to 1997, it struggled to succeed in the market, particularly when Jobs left and in the face of escalating competition from other behemoths like IBM, who dominated the PC market (Elmansy, R., 2016). Apple experienced a lot of difficulties during this time, including:

- Unstable strategy as a result of switching executive teams.
- Unclear competitive strategy, especially since IBM entered the PC industry.
- Uncertainty around the sale of OS licenses that would pit the business against the Windows operating system.
- Numerous unsuccessful products (such as the *Newton PDA*) and a small number of profitable ones (such as the *PowerBook*).
- Products with no distinguishing features.
- Customers are confused and uncertain as to the company's future.

4.2.1 Redesigning the iPhone

Apple used design-thinking to improve the user experience of the iPhone. They conducted extensive user research to understand pain points and areas of improvement. Through this process, they identified issues such as difficulty in accessing certain features and a lack of customization options. As a result, Apple introduced features like *Control Center* for easy access to settings, *Siri* for voice commands, and the ability to customize the home screen layout. These design changes aim to make the iPhone more intuitive and personalized for users.

4.2.2 Creating the Apple Watch

Apple applied design-thinking principles when creating the Apple Watch. They conducted user research to understand the needs and preferences of potential users. Through this process, they discovered that users wanted a device that seamlessly integrated with their daily activities and provided health and fitness tracking. As a result, Apple designed the Apple Watch with features like activity tracking, heart-rate monitoring, and seamless integration with other Apple devices—these design choices aimed to create a wearable device that met the needs and desires of users.

4.2.3 Redesigning the MacBook Pro

Apple addressed customer concerns and feedback with the MacBook Pro by utilizing design-thinking. To comprehend problems like limited connectivity options and upgradability, they carried out user research. Apple introduced features like *Touch Bar* for customizable shortcuts and *Thunderbolt 3* ports for more connectivity options through this process. The goal of these design adjustments is to provide users with more flexibility and productivity.

4.2.4 Improving the Apple Store Experience

Apple employed design-thinking principles to improve the overall experience at Apple Stores. They researched to understand customer preferences and pain points. Through this process, Apple redesigned store layouts, introduced features like *Today at Apple* sessions for educational experiences, and improved customer service interactions. These design changes aim to create a more engaging and personalized experience for customers.

Apple is now among the industry leaders when it comes to innovation, and this wouldn't have been possible without the business embracing design-thinking. Apple has been able to produce products that are not just aesthetically pleasing but also practical and user-friendly by embracing design-thinking. By consistently coming up with new ideas and refining their products in response to customer input, they have been able to stay one step ahead of the competition.

4.3 IDEO

IDEO is a well-known international design consultancy that uses design-thinking techniques. They have designed a new shopping cart for a large retailer, among other projects. The designers at IDEO watched and spoke with customers to learn about their dissatisfaction with current shopping carts. After that, they developed a new cart that addressed these issues through iteration and prototyping, making shopping more efficient and pleasurable. Here are some case studies that show how IDEO applied the concepts of design-thinking:

4.3.1 Redesigning the Shopping Cart

A major US grocery store chain approached IDEO to improve the shopping cart experience. IDEO's designers began by empathizing with shoppers and observing their behaviors and frustrations. They discovered issues such as maneuverability, shopping behavior, child safety, and maintenance costs. The cases they take into consideration involve shopping carts that are frequently swept away by the wind at a high speed, raising questions about the safety of the children riding in the carts as well as pedestrians in the parking lot or grocery store. A team of designers considered these issues when creating prototypes of new grocery cart designs, and their concepts were amazing.

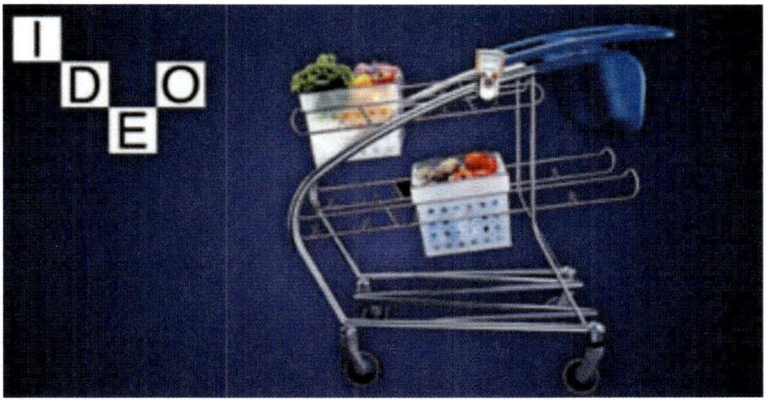

Figure 4.1: IDEO Shopping Cart Project

One group offered a shopping cart with a built-in scanner to scan items that are added while shopping and another attached a speaker device to the cart so that customers can interact with store staff. The goal was to take into account all group designs and combine them into a single, final prototype that functions as the best shopping cart possible (Chui, C, 2016). The new cart design not only improved the shopping experience but also increased sales for the grocery store.

4.3.2 Designing a Better Hospital Experience

IDEO worked with a hospital to improve the patient experience in the emergency department (UserTesting, 2022). The IDEO team began by imagining themselves in the patient's shoes. By having one of their team members act as a patient in the hospital, they were able to uncover something that was both evident and ignored. They began by playing a six-minute video clip of the ceiling in a patient's room before presenting their findings to the hospital executives. Initially, the executives were perplexed and had no idea what they were seeing. The IDEO team went on to describe the video's purpose.

The idea was that a patient had a very unpleasant experience when they were forced to lie in bed all day, starting at the ceiling. The executives were able to grasp "*a blinding glimpse of the bloody obvious*" after watching the video clip, according to Paul Bennett, Chief Creative Officer at IDEO (UserTesting, 2019).

It dawned on them to view the patient experience from the patient's perspective rather than the organization's, and they acted upon it right away.

They came to understand that enhancing the patient experience did not require significantly altering the system. Rather, the focus should be on taking small actions that have a significant effect. IDEO then began ideation and prototyping, and they swiftly put four minor changes into practice:

- Added decorations to the ceilings to improve aesthetics.
- Whiteboards were placed on one wall of each patient's room so that visitors could leave notes for the patient.
- Made the hospital hallway floors one color and style different from the floors in the patient rooms. This gave patients the impression that they were in their own space and marked the change between public and private space.
- Rear-view mirrors were installed on hospital gurneys so that patients could see the person they were talking to while being wheeled around by a nurse or doctor.

4.3.3 Redesign the ATM experience

The IDEO design team began by conducting interviews and watching customers use ATMs at bank branches in Spain, Mexico, and the United States, including BBVA (short for Banco Bilbao Vizcaya Argentaria). The group also looked into self-service transactions at train ticket kiosks, supermarket checkout lanes, and gas pumps. One of the things they discovered was that when people in the line could see over their shoulders while they were making purchases, it made them uncomfortable. IDEO and BBVA decided to turn the machine 90 degrees so that a privacy screen blocked onlooker view (Brand, T. F., 2010). In addition, the new design include features such as personalized greetings, customizable options for frequently used transactions, and a simplified interface. The redesigned ATMs were rolled out in select locations in the United States in 2017.

4.3.4 Designing a New Voting System

IDEO designers collaborated closely with LA County employees to develop a voting system that takes into account the particular complexities of the constituency's voter base, such as its extremely diverse population and its numerous election laws and policies. Designers needed to create a voting system that would be helpful and accessible to voters of all ages and backgrounds, including those who are visually impaired, use wheelchairs, have learning disabilities, are not tech-savvy, or speak languages other than English (Ideo, 2016).

The objective was to design a voting process that voters feel comfortable with, balancing their emotional and practical needs, and to create a system that can be modified over time. One device will be available for everyone to use.

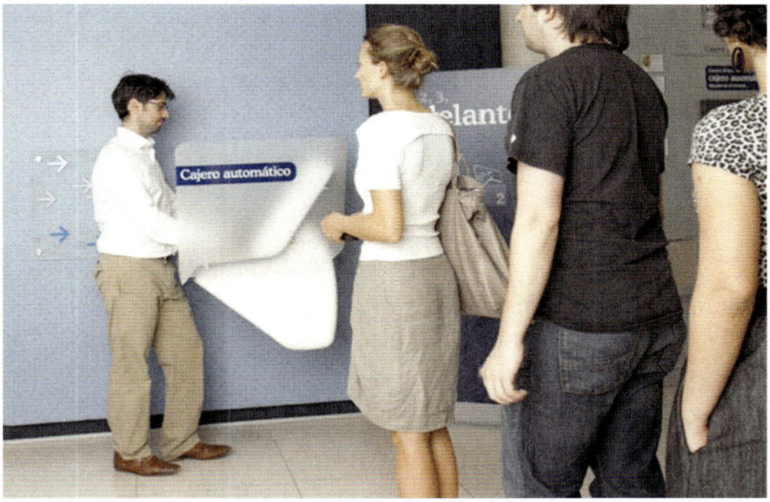

Figure 4.2: Redesign the ATM Experience

The resultant prototype is a voting device that can be customized for various user experiences. It was created in partnership with Cambridge Consultants and Digital Foundry. By navigating through various screens that display lists of candidates and ballot measures, a touch screen makes it simple for any voter to complete the ballot.

Voters with visual impairments or reading difficulties can navigate their options with the touch of a few easy buttons on an audio controller interface. Additionally, using the same machine, voters can select their preferred language to read the ballot in: Spanish, Chinese, Korean, or any of the 11 languages the county supports. They get a printed paper ballot that fits into an integrated ballot box after they tap in their choices on the device.

4.3.5 Reimagining School Lunch

The San Francisco Unified School District and IDEO collaborated in 2013 to update the elementary school lunch program. The IDEO team conducted interviews with students in schools. When they asked children how they would like to make their lunch experience better, they frequently received the following response: "If you just started serving ice cream, from the minute we get in here until the time we leave, that would be perfect." The team realized that lunch was about more than just food when they watched children eat. Lunch is an opportunity to socialize. Lunch is the first opportunity the kids get to spend time with their friends after spending the entire morning in their classrooms.

Some children even went so far as to skip lunch to hang out with their friends for longer. Given that kids do not care about lunch, IDEO realized they should be designing an extraordinary experience around hanging out with friends rather than an extraordinary experience around lunch. Getting rid of waiting lines, taking the food out from behind the counters, and serving lunch to the kids in a family-style manner so that they can enter, sit down at a table, and begin spending time with friends right away. The fact that fruits and vegetables are served first makes the children eat them because they are hungry and nothing else on the table was one of the best innovations.

In these case studies, IDEO demonstrates the application of design-thinking principles such as empathy, ideation, prototyping, and iteration. By deeply understanding the needs and desires of users, collaborating with stakeholders, and rapidly testing and refining solutions, IDEO was able to create innovative and impactful designs.

4.4 IBM

IBM has applied design-thinking to enhance its internal processes and culture. They established *IBM Design*, a program that trains employees in design-thinking methodologies and encourages cross-functional collaboration. By incorporating design-thinking into its organizational DNA, IBM has been able to foster innovation, improve user experiences, and create products and services that better meet the needs of its clients.

IBM developed an enterprise design-thinking framework with an emphasis on user outcomes, especially to support diverse teams working together on larger enterprise-level projects. Understanding, exploring, prototyping, and validating ideas with users are all part of the iterative process of enterprise design-thinking, which is similar to traditional design-thinking.

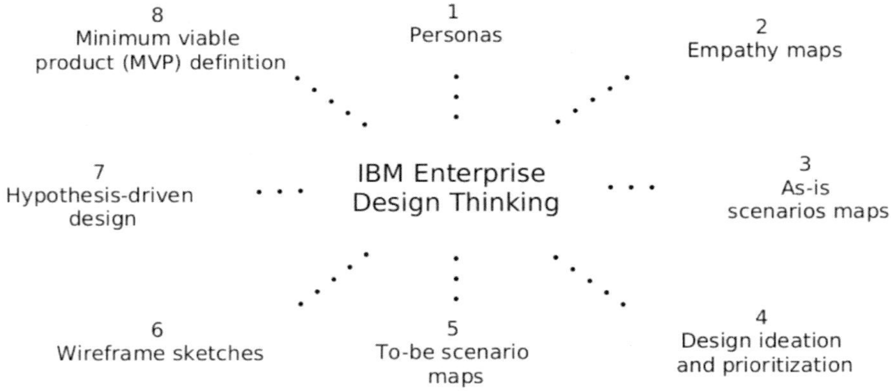

Figure 4.3: Components of Enterprise Design-Thinking

According to Pesot, J. and Plantenberg, S. (2023) enterprise design-thinking involves several components, including:

- **Persona:** designers use a variety of sources, such as forums, surveys, in-person observations, and interviews, to obtain data. Following this, the data is completed into an outline that describes one or more personas—specific people who stand in for the intended audience.
- **Empathy Maps**: after the creation of personas, their thoughts, feelings, words, and actions are recorded.
- **As-is Scenarios Maps:** record every concern and issue the personas attributes.
- **Design Ideation and Prioritization:** brainstorming to come up with as many ideas as possible to thrill the target audience and solve their problems. After generating these ideas, the next step is to group them and assess which ones offer the most potential for impact and success.
- **To-be Scenario Maps**: explain what will happen in the future when strong design concepts are adopted.
- **Wireframe Sketches:** making a series of low-fidelity sketches with different options can be helpful at times.
- **Hypothesis-Driven Design:** designing and delivering a set of measurable and testable hypotheses is a fundamental component of Enterprise design-thinking.
- **Minimum Viable Product (MVP) Definition:** based on the hypothesis development, the smallest scale product that can be rapidly produced to aid in the learning process, and allow designers to assess their work.

IBM has utilized enterprise design-thinking in various case studies to drive innovation and create user-centric solutions. Here are a few examples:

4.4.1 Generative AI (GenAI)

Every call a consumer makes to a call center presents the business with a chance to learn. However, important information is lost when call center representatives are too busy to review automatically recorded transactions that have already been logged. Using Generative AI (GenAI), IBM has been able to solve a problem for a major European telco. The agents in the telco's call center were too busy to go through the transcripts of their earlier interactions with customers. There were gaps in the organization's CRM (Customer Relationship Management) due to incomplete customer conversation recording. These transcripts were hardly used because they were long and incomplete (Cushman, D., 2023).

According to HFS research, one of the first areas that generative artificial intelligence (GenAI) will impact is customer operations, which includes customer service functions. IBM's solution made use of two large language models (LLMs), also referred to as GenAI foundation models.

- In the first LLM instance, IBM used GenAI's natural language understanding capabilities to create automatic call summarization. This involved using the transcription of the conversation to create a more readable summary that was broken down into three or four bullet points. The LLM was also taught to recognize and extract important subjects.
- The second LLM uses conversation analysis to identify attrition risk in customer interactions. It examines sentiment, emotion analysis, and references to the telco's rivals. The analysis can determine when to make counteroffers or give information to comprehend the reasons behind customer attrition.

Apart from these, IBM applied design-thinking principles to develop many solutions, as follows:

- **IBM Watson:** IBM applied design-thinking principles to develop Watson, an AI-powered cognitive computing system.
- **IBM Design Language:** IBM implemented design-thinking to create a unified design language across its products and services.
- **IBM Cloud Garage:** IBM's Cloud Garage is a design-thinking-based approach to help clients accelerate their cloud adoption and innovation.
- **IBM Design Studios:** IBM established design studios worldwide to foster a culture of design-thinking within the organization.

Overall, IBM's use of design-thinking in these case studies demonstrates its commitment to understanding users' needs, empathizing with their experiences, and creating solutions that are human-centered and impactful.

4.5 Stanford d.school

Stanford University's d.school is known for its application of design-thinking across disciplines. One example is their collaboration with the healthcare industry. By using design-thinking methods, they identified the need for improved patient experiences and developed solutions such as redesigned hospital rooms, streamlined processes, and innovative medical devices.

The Stanford d.school (officially known as the Hasso Plattner Institute of Design at Stanford University) is a renowned design-thinking institute that has been instrumental in introducing design-thinking methodologies to various industries. Here are some case studies that demonstrate how the d.school has used design-thinking to solve complex problems:

4.5.1 Redesigning the Emergency Room Experience

The d.school redesigned the ER experience for patients in partnership with Stanford Hospital and Clinics. Finding methods to enhance the hospital's emergency department patient experience was their main objective. They role-played with patients and their families during the exercise to simulate what it's like to be in the frequently chaotic environment of an emergency room. Interviews, tabletop exercises, and modeling real work routines in the suggested floor plans of the nursing units that needed to be redesigned were all part of the seven-month process (Wykes, S., 2016).

The first day of the class produced an extensive amount of data that would guide the second prototyping day: finding certain themes wasn't difficult at all. Patients wanted assurances that communication was occurring between their healthcare providers and that they were routinely provided with information to help them make sense of what was happening. They asserted that clear and efficient communication would significantly lessen their elevated fear and anxiety.

4.5.2 The Wallet Project

A design challenge that asks students to create a wallet for a specific user, taking into account their needs and preferences. This is a brief practical introduction to design-thinking. "The Wallet Project is a fast-paced, ninety-minute project that goes through a full design cycle (plus debrief). Students work in pairs, sharing information about their wallets as they brainstorm and create an innovative idea that is both "useful and meaningful" for their partner (Vermijlen, B, 2016). The structure beautifully reflects the 4 D's of design-thinking, as shown in Figure 4.4.

The *Double Diamond* is based on the frame innovation approach developed by Kees Dorst, University of Technology Professor of Design Innovation. The design process, according to his approach, can be divided into problem space and solution space. The problem space is the stage at which designers investigate the problem, including its complexities, and conclude with a clear definition of the problem. It is the location of the majority of unique design characteristics and values, such as creativity and uncertainty. The solution space is the second stage, where ideas are generated, visualized, and prototypes tested. The final product is created and delivered to the end user at the end of this stage.

A couple of nice examples of what the class came up with are: a wallet that has a removable compartment that fits into a woman's bra, allowing the user to party without having to be concerned about losing their essentials, a wallet with a removable part that contains precious memories that may be left behind when the owner is going to a party.

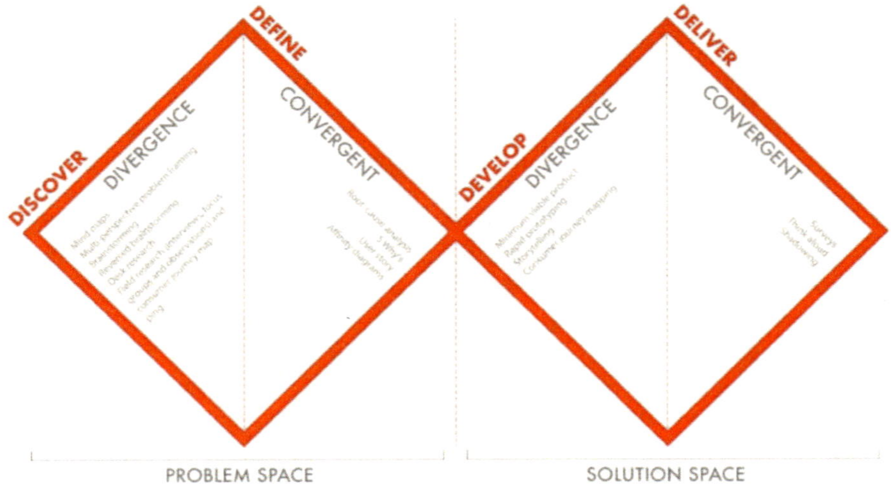

Figure 4.4: The Double Diamond design-thinking Process (adopted from the Design Council)

Overall, these case studies demonstrate how the d.school uses design-thinking methodologies to understand the needs and pain points of users, develop innovative solutions, and create a positive impact in various industries.

4.6 Ford

Ford has used design-thinking to reimagine the car-buying experience with their *FordPass* platform. They researched to understand the pain points of car buyers, such as the complexity of the purchasing process and the lack of transparency. Using design-thinking principles, they created an app that allows users to browse inventory, schedule test drives, and even complete the entire car-buying process online. This innovative approach has helped Ford differentiate itself in the competitive automotive industry (Ranjan, S., 2024).

- **FordPass:** is a mobile app that allows Ford owners to access a range of services, including remote start, vehicle location tracking, and maintenance alerts. The app was developed to make it easier for Ford owners to manage their vehicles and stay connected to their cars.
- **SYNC 3:** is Ford's infotainment system, which was designed to be more intuitive and user-friendly than previous versions. The system features a touchscreen interface, voice recognition, and integration with popular apps like Apple CarPlay and Android Auto.
- **Ford Co-Pilot360:** is a suite of driver-assist technologies that help drivers stay safe on the road. The system includes features like

lane-keeping assist, automatic emergency braking, and adaptive cruise control. These features were developed to reduce accidents and make driving less stressful for Ford customers.

- **FordPass Charging Network:** is a network of charging stations for electric vehicles (EVs). The network was developed to make it easier for Ford EV owners to find charging stations and plan their trips accordingly.
- **Ford GoRide Health:** is a non-emergency medical transportation service that was developed in partnership with healthcare providers. The service is designed to provide reliable and affordable transportation for patients who need to get to medical appointments. This solution was developed to improve access to healthcare for people who might otherwise struggle to get to appointments.

Ford's approach to design thinking goes beyond mere jargon; it's a practical, industry-inspiring model. By focusing on real people and real problems, Ford has sustained its success. This focus has allowed them to design cars that resonate with consumers, foster a workforce aligned with business goals, and navigate the complexities of the global market effectively.

4.7 Conclusion

These case studies demonstrate how design-thinking can be applied across various industries to solve complex problems, improve user experiences, and drive innovation.

References

Brand, T. F. 2010. Atm 2.0: the future of self-service. https://thefinancialbrand.com/news/banking-technology/bbva-ideo-atm-of-the-future-12706/. (Accessed: Accessed: January 16, 2024)

Chaturvedi, N. 2020. How apple used design thinking? https://medium.com/macoclock/how-apple-used-design-thinking-38afb6770a6. (Accessed: July 27, 2020)

Cheng, V. 2018. Airbnb case study: designing to facilitate the booking process. https://medium.com/@vcmimi1998/airbnb-case-study-designing-to-facilitate-the-booking-process-33731280b8c8. (Accessed: July 11, 2023).

Chui, C. 2016. Design thinking. https://medium.com/@claudiachui/design-thinking-27b2aaba6688. (Accessed: December 27, 2022) .

Cushman, D. 2023. IBM uses genai to help euro telco call-center team work better. https://www.hfsresearch.com/research/ibm-uses-genai-to-help-euro-telco-call-center-team-work-better/. (Accessed: December 31, 2023).

Ellis, S. 2015. How design thinking transformed airbnb from a failing startup to a billion dollar business. Retrieved July, 14, 2016.

Elmansy, R. 2016. Design thinking case study: innovation at apple. https://www.designorate.com/design-thinking-case-study-innovation-at-apple/. (Accessed: Juy 13, 2023).

Enginess. 2023. Unlocking innovation: design thinking case studies and tools. https://www.enginess.io/insights/Unlocking-Innovatio-Design-Thinking-Case-Studies-and-Tools. (Accessed: December 28, 2022)

FasterCapital. 2024. Ultimate faq:airbnb, what, how, why, when. https://fastercapital.com/content/Ultimate-FAQ-Airbnb--What--How--Why--When.html. (Accessed: October 26, 2024).

Ideo. 2016. A new way to vote for the people of los angeles. https://www.ideo.com/works/a-new-way-to-vote-for-the-people-of-los-angeles. (Accessed: November 30, 2023).

Pesot, J. and Plantenberg, S. 2023. Enterprise design thinking. https://www.ibm.com/garage/method/practices/think/enterprise-design-thinking/. (Accessed: December 30, 2023).

Ranjan, S. 2024. Design thinking: Ford's path to excellence. https://medium.com/@saketranjan126/design-thinking-fords-path-to-excellence-591e3de74dc4. (Accessed: October 25, 2024).

User Testing. 2019. IDEO's human centered design process: How to make things people love. https://www.usertesting.com/blog/how-ideo-uses-customer-insights-to-design-innovative-products-users-love. (Accessed: January 12, 2024).

UserTesting. 2022. Ideo's human centered design process. https://www.usertesting.com/resources/topics/ideos-human-centered-design-process. (Accessed: December, 25, 2023).

Vermijlen, B. 2016. Design thinking exercise: the wallet project—bart vermijlen. https://www.bartvermijlen.com/design-thinking-exercise-wallet-project/. (Accessed: December 31, 2023).

Walsh, C., Saxena, D. and Muzellec, L. 2020. Airbnb: Managing trust and safety on a platform business. The Irish Journal of Management. 39(2): 126–134. Retrieved from https://doi.org/10.2478/ijm-2020-0004 doi: doi:10.2478/ijm-2020-0004.

Wykes, S. 2016. Design thinking as a way to improve patient experience. https://med.stanford.edu/news/all-news/2016/06/design-thinking-as-a-way-to-improve-patient-experience.html?microsite=news&tab=news. (Accessed: December 31, 2023).

Chapter 5

Tools and Techniques

Design-thinking employs tools and technologies to aid in the processes of ideation, prototyping, and testing. Design-thinking is a method of problem-solving that stresses empathy, creativity, and iteration. A variety of tools and technologies are employed to create ideas, illustrate concepts, and test prototypes to properly apply this technique. From identifying customer demands to designing and testing solutions, Lewrick, Michael and Link, Patrick and Leifer, Larry (2018) offer useful tools and methods for each step of the process. Additionally, they provide case studies and examples from a variety of industries to show how Design-thinking may be used in many settings. Liedtka, Jeanne and Ogilvie, Tim (2011) provides a toolkit for managers to use throughout the Design-thinking process, from identifying opportunities to prototyping and testing solutions. There are several tools and techniques commonly used in Design-thinking. Some of the most popular ones include:

- Empathize Tools—Root cause, Personas, CJM, and EM
- Define Tools—Problem Statement, POV
- Ideate Tools—Brainstorming, Mind Map, SWOT, Sketching
- Prototype Tools—Paper, Lego, Digital, Wizard
- Test Tools—User, Usability, A/B, Accessibility, Performance
- Future Tools—AR, VR, AI, Collaboration, 3D Printing

5.1 Tools and Techniques for Practicing Empathy

Although extensively discussed in the previous chapter, data for empathy research may be gathered through focus groups, interviews, observation, and other methods, it was not explained how this research is carried out or how the data is arranged to provide an appropriate context for future solutions. To obtain an understanding of the information, some tools are covered in this section.

5.1.1 Root Cause Analysis Tool

Design thinkers use this technique to find the root cause of the problem. As previously discussed, a variety of techniques are used to collect data from users. During the data collection phase, the root cause analysis technique is employed to elicit the necessary information from users. Tools like the 5 Whys Technique, Cause-Effect Diagrams, and Failure Mode and Effects Analysis are designed to help investigate the root causes of a problem, which can contribute to finding the correct solution (Elmansy, R., 2023).

5.1.1.1 5 Whys Technique

The 5 Whys Technique is a way of problem-solving that involves asking *why* frequently. It is a means of promptly identifying the underlying cause of a problem. Throughout the 1930s, Japanese industrialist, inventor, and founder of Toyota Industries, Sakichi Toyoda, developed the 5 Whys Technique. Toyota has been using it to solve issues since the 1970s when it first gained popularity. Pojasek (2000) proposed four steps of the 5 Whys Techniques as follows:

- **Assemble a Team and Define the Problem:** gather together people who are familiar with the specifics of the problem, and with the process that design thinkers are trying to improve.
- **Ask the First *Why*?:** a member of the design team inquires as to the reason behind the issue. It is possible this elicits three or four responses. Every response must be recorded.
- **Ask *Why?* Four More Times:** For the preceding answers, pose four more consecutive why questions. Keep all of the solutions close to the parents. Investigate every response that seems plausible. When asking *why* no longer yields useful answers, the team can identify the underlying cause of the issue and move forward.
- **Investigate the Primary Cause(s) and Track Interventions:** after at least one root cause has been found, the next step is to discuss and decide on the countermeasures that will stop the issue from happening again. Monitoring closely the extent to which the countermeasures reduce or eliminate the original issue is necessary.

To understand the 5 whys analysis, let's look at an example of a restaurant where customers are complaining about the quality of the food. The 5 whys analysis is shown in Figure 5.1. Employee training is the root cause of the issue. To improve food quality and customer satisfaction, the restaurant could greatly benefit from funding employee training initiatives to make sure that the staff in the kitchen follows recipes precisely and prepares food correctly.

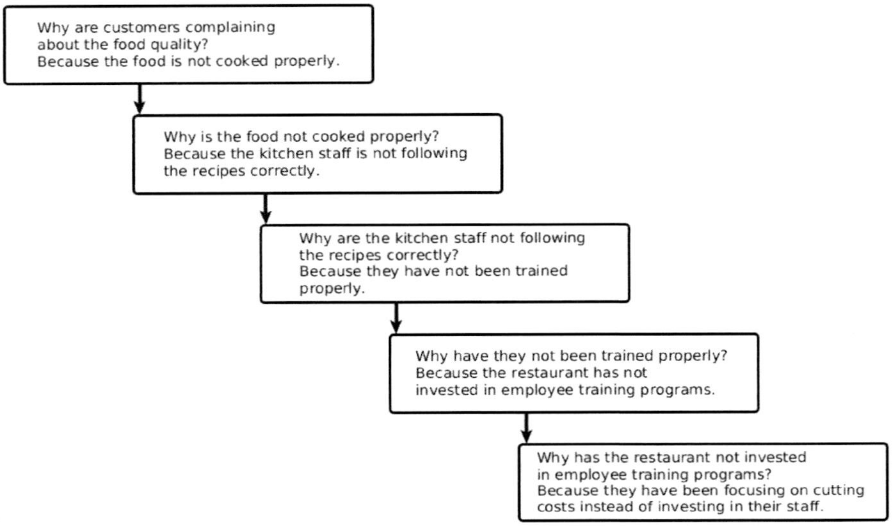
Why are customers complaining about the food quality?
Because the food is not cooked properly.
Why is the food not cooked properly?
Because the kitchen staff is not following the recipes correctly.
Why are the kitchen staff not following the recipes correctly?
Because they have not been trained properly.
Why have they not been trained properly?
Because the restaurant has not invested in employee training programs.
Why has the restaurant not invested in employee training programs?
Because they have been focusing on cutting costs instead of investing in their staff.

Figure 5.1: 5 Why Analysis

The 5 Whys method is simple yet effective for determining the root cause of a problem. It aids in the identification of underlying issues that may not be immediately apparent and allows for the development of targeted solutions.

5.1.1.2 Cause-Effect Diagram

This is another tool that is used in empathy research. A cause-and-effect diagram, also known as an Ishikawa diagram or a fishbone diagram, is a visual tool used to identify the possible causes of a problem. It is called a fishbone diagram because it looks like the skeleton of a fish, with the problem statement at the head of the fish and the potential causes branching off like the bones of the fish. Dr. Kaoru Ishikawa, a Japanese quality control expert, is credited with developing the fishbone diagram to assist employees in avoiding solutions that only address the symptoms of a much larger problem.

Lewis, S. (2020), provided some instructions for creating a fishbone diagram. Usually, fishbone diagrams are created during a team meeting on a flipchart or whiteboard. Teams can proceed with the following steps to create the diagram once an issue has been identified that needs further investigation:

- The problem is listed in statement form, and a box is drawn around it to create the fish's head. After that, a head-pointing horizontal arrow is drawn across the page. This is the fish's backbone.

- Next, a minimum of four comprehensive *causes* are recognized as potential contributors to the problem. Methods, skills, equipment, staff, materials, environment, and measurements are a few general categories to start with. After that, arrows are drawn from these causes to branch off from the spine, creating the fish's initial bones.
- Team members can benefit greatly from coming up with any supporting details that can help each overarching cause. To keep the conversation focused, this usually entails using some form of questioning techniques, like the 4Ps (Policies, Procedures, People, and Plant) or the 5 Whys. These contributing elements are listed in order of decreasing distance from their respective causes.
- Once the fundamental causes of the issue have been found, the process of dissecting each cause is carried out once more. The group then examines the diagram to determine a conclusion and decide on the next step of action.

This is an example of how a fishbone diagram can be used to improve customer satisfaction in a restaurant. The problem in this case is poor food quality.

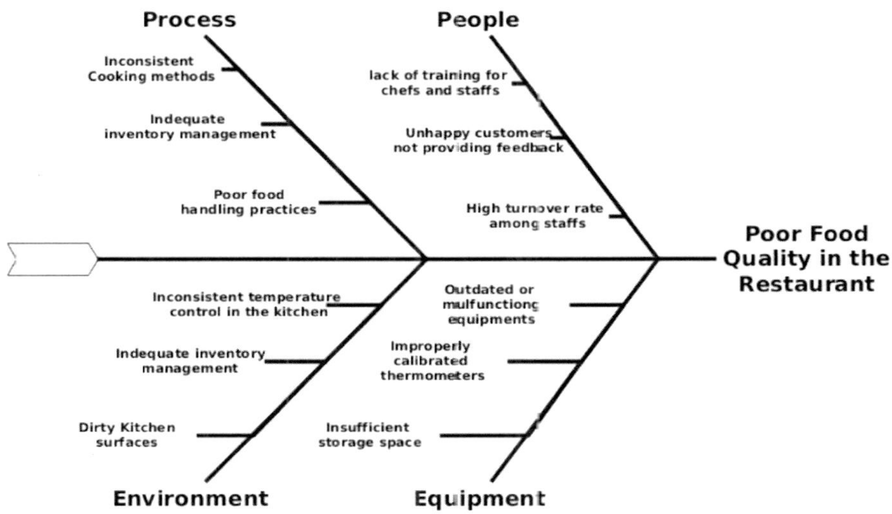

Figure 5.2: Fishbone Diagram

By using a fishbone diagram to identify and analyze the possible causes of poor food quality in a restaurant, design thinkers can develop targeted solutions to address the root causes and improve the overall quality of the food and customer experience.

5.1.2 User Personas

User personas are most widely used in empathy research. User personas are fictional representations of the ideal customers or users of a product or service. They are created based on research and data about the target audience and are used to guide the design and development of products that meet their needs and preferences. User personas typically include information about demographics, behavior patterns, goals, motivations, and pain points.

To create user personas, design thinkers and researchers start by gathering data about the target audience. This might include conducting surveys, interviews, or focus groups; analyzing website analytics or social media data; or conducting ethnographic research to observe users in their natural environments.

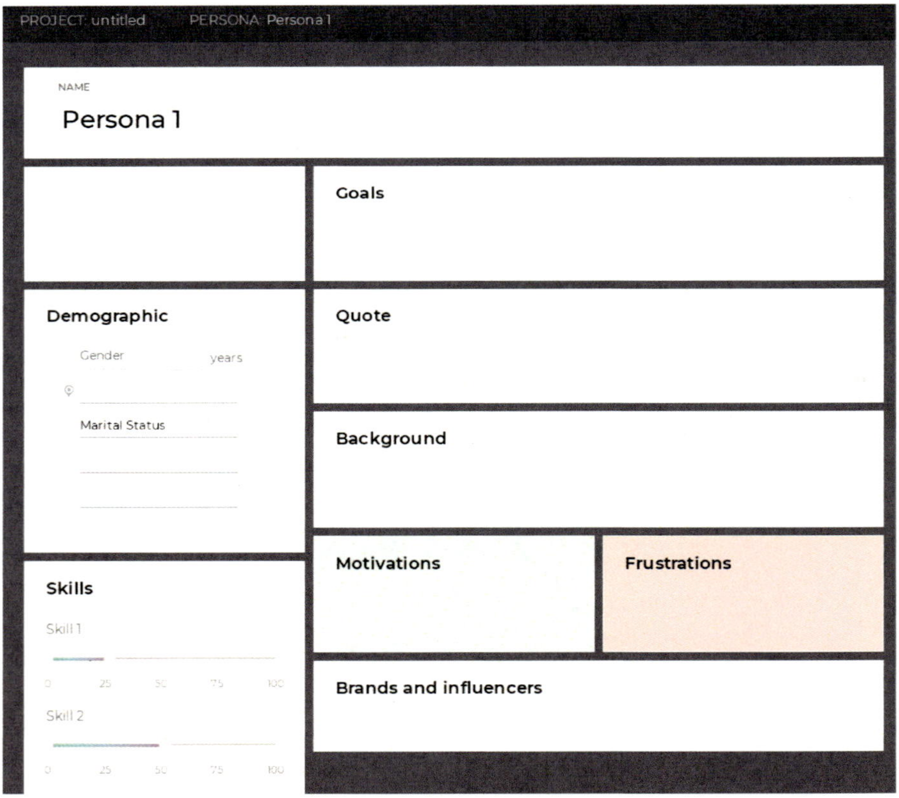

Figure 5.3: Persona

McCay, A. (2023a) proposed some of the steps to create the persons using uxpressia website.

- **Step One:** research. Data is gathered through a variety of research methods, including focus groups, interviews, observation, and more, as covered in previous chapters.
- **Step Two:** developing the persona seeks to segment the audience. It is imperative to remember that a single persona cannot serve as a representative of the whole clientele. It must consist of a significant subset of clients with similar characteristics, requirements, goals, and behaviors.
- **Step Three:** deciding the layout. Depending on the persona type and purpose, layouts can vary. The persona has a flexible structure. For instance, whereas some concentrate on behavioral characteristics, others may represent demographic information.
- **Step Four:** set demographic information. This includes basic information such as age, gender, income, education level, and geographic location.
- **Step Five:** describe the Persona's background. It can be of great benefit to document all available background information. Keeping in mind that even the smallest detail can reveal something insightful for their company. Conversely, extraneous details that could confuse and clutter the page should be avoided. There should be two objectives for this step: to inspire empathy and to provide insightful and useful information.
- **Step Six:** define the persona's goals. This includes information about what users hope to achieve by using the product or service, such as saving time, increasing productivity, or improving their health.
- **Step Seven:** define motivations and frustrations. This includes information about the problems or frustrations when using the product or service, such as difficulty navigating the interface or slow load times.
- **Step Eight:** Add other ingredients. At this stage, persona is almost complete, but there is still plenty of room for enhancement.

  In UXPressia's Personas tool, designers can enrich their Persona by adding a variety of sections to paint a more detailed picture of their real or ideal customer. Consider adding elements like skills, key touchpoints, the technology their Persona uses, quotes, and more to make it as comprehensive as possible.

User personas are typically presented in a visual format that includes a name, photo, and brief description of characteristics. Developers often use them to guide decisions about product features, user interface design, and marketing strategies. By creating user personas, teams can better understand the needs and preferences of their target audience and design products that meet those needs more effectively. O'Donoghue, J. (2023), gives the advantages and disadvantages of personas as shown in Table 5.1.

Table 5.1: Advantages and Disadvantages of Personss

Advantages	Disadvantages
Personas assist businesses in understanding their customers' needs, preferences, behaviors, and motivations.	Personas are based on assumptions and generalizations that may not accurately represent all customers
Personas serve as helpful reminders of research findings throughout the rest of the design process, ensuring that designers stay on track and meet the user needs.	Persona development can be time-consuming and costly, especially if businesses conduct extensive research to gather data and insights.
Personas help design thinkers stay focused on the most critical aspects of the user's journey by emphasizing the key elements that matter most to the user.	Personas may quickly become outdated as customer needs and preferences change. Businesses must continuously update and refine their personas for them to remain relevant and effective.

5.1.3 Customer Journey Map (CJM)

This technique involves mapping out the user's journey from start to finish and identifying pain points and opportunities for improvement. A customer journey map visualizes and understands customers' experiences as they interact with a product or service. It involves creating a step-by-step map of the customer's journey, from initial awareness to post-purchase follow-up. Journey mapping helps businesses gain insights into customer behavior, pain points, and opportunities for improvement. McCay, A. (2023b) suggested the process of creating a customer journey map that typically involves the following steps:

- **Step 1:** defining the persona is the first step in creating a customer journey map.
- **Step 2:** once the persona is created, it is necessary to identify the stages of the customer journey map. For example, *Aware, Research, Arrival, Order, Eat, Leave, Feedback, and Return.*

    1. ***Awareness:*** customers become aware of the brand or product.
    2. ***Research:*** customers start to research and evaluate the product or service.
    3. ***Purchase:*** customers decide to purchase the product or service.
    4. ***Onboarding:*** after the purchase, customers need to be onboarded and introduced to the product or service.

5. ***Usage:*** how customers use the product or service and their experience with it.
6. ***Support:*** customers may need support during their usage of the product or service.
7. ***Loyalty:*** how satisfied customers are with the product or service and are theylikely to become repeat customers or advocates for the brand.
8. ***Advocacy:*** customers become advocates for the brand and recommend it to others.

- **Step 3:** setting customer goals: There are several reasons why it's a good idea to set customer goals at every stage: facilitates design thinkers' comprehension of how their business goals coincide with those of their customers and more comprehensively serve the needs of customers and win their loyalty by assisting them in reaching all of their goals.
- **Step 4:** defining touchpoints: Touchpoints are encounters that happen between the business and customers. Here are examples of touchpoints for a customer journey map of a pizza order:

  1. ***Awareness:*** the customer sees an advertisement for a pizza delivery service on social media.
  2. ***Research:*** the customer visits the website to browse the menu, read reviews, and compare prices.
  3. ***Purchase:*** the customer places an order online or over the phone and pays for the pizza.
  4. ***Onboarding:*** the customer receives an email or text message confirming the order and providing an estimated delivery time.
  5. ***Usage:*** the customer receives the pizza and enjoys eating it.
  6. ***Support:*** if there are any issues with the order, the customer can contact customer support for assistance.
  7. ***Loyalty:*** if the customer is satisfied with the pizza and delivery experience, they may become a repeat customer.
  8. ***Advocacy:*** the customer may leave a positive review on the website or recommend the pizza delivery service to friends and family.

  Defining all the touchpoints is critical because each touchpoint leaves a distinct impression, and the main goal is to keep it up to the mark.
- **Step 5:** problems and ideas. Explore problems users might have when using the service. Here are some potential problems and ideas for each stage of the customer journey map for a pizza order:

1. In the awareness stage, customers are perhaps unaware of the existence of the pizza delivery service. The idea is to use targeted advertising on social media and search engines to reach out to potential customers in the area.
2. In the research stage, the customer may have difficulty navigating the website or finding the information they need. The idea is to simplify the website design and provide clear menus, pricing, and reviews to make the decision-making process.
3. In the purchase stage, the customer may encounter technical issues or have difficulty completing the payment process. The idea is to ensure the website is user-friendly and secure and offer multiple payment options to accommodate different preferences.
4. In the onboarding stage, the estimated delivery time may be inaccurate, or the customer may not receive confirmation of their order. The idea is to use real-time tracking and notifications to keep the customer informed about their order status and expected delivery time.
5. In the usage stage, the pizza may arrive cold or damaged, or it may not meet the customer's expectations. The idea is to ensure the pizza is prepared and delivered on time and offer quality guarantees or refunds for unsatisfied customers.
6. In the support stage, the customer may encounter issues with their order or have questions about the service. The idea is to offer responsive and helpful customer support via phone, email, or chat to address any concerns or issues that arise.
7. In the loyalty stage, the customer may not feel incentivized to return or become a loyal customer. The idea is to offer loyalty programs, discounts, or personalized recommendations based on the customer's past orders to encourage repeat business.
8. In the advocacy stage, the customer may not feel motivated to leave a positive review or recommend the service to others. The idea is to encourage satisfied customers to share their experiences on social media or review sites and offer incentives or rewards for referrals or positive feedback.

The customer journey map is a process that requires ongoing monitoring and refinement to ensure that the customer experience remains optimal. By understanding the customer journey and identifying pain points and opportunities, businesses can improve customer satisfaction, increase loyalty, and drive revenue growth.

5.1.4 Empathy Mapping

This tool helps design thinkers understand the needs, thoughts, and emotions of users by creating a visual representation of their experiences. Empathy mapping is a tool used in design-thinking to help teams understand the needs and perspectives of their users or customers. It involves creating a visual representation of the user's experience and emotions, which can then be used to inform the design of products or services.

To create an empathy map, teams typically start by identifying the user or customer they want to understand (Goulbourne, Catherine Pear, 2019). Generally, they then divide a whiteboard or piece of paper into four quadrants, each representing a different aspect of the user's experience. Nowadays, online tools like uxpressia, provide the platform to design empathy maps with more quadrants.

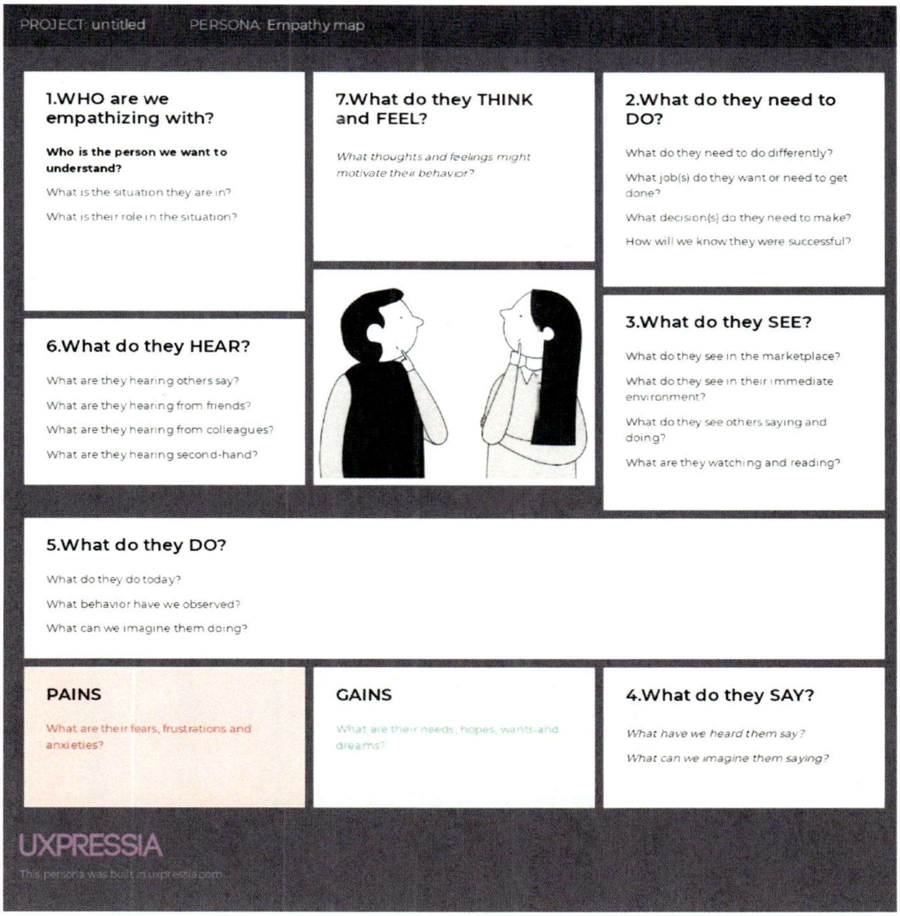

Figure 5.4: Empathy Map

- *Who are we empathizing with?*: this quadrant contains information that design thinkers should be aware of, including the people they want to understand, the situations users find themselves in, and their involvement in those situations. It involves placing design thinkers in the shoes of users and experiencing what users are experiencing.
- *What do they need to do?*: this quadrant contains observations about what users should do differently, tasks that users need to complete or want to accomplish, choices that users must make, and ways that designers will be able to determine if their efforts were successful.
- *What do they SEE?*: this quadrant observes what users see in the store, what users see in their immediate surroundings, what users observe other users saying and doing, and what users watch and read.
- *What do they SAY?*: This quadrant captures the user's words and phrases, such as quotes from interviews or feedback from surveys. It helps teams understand the user's language and vocabulary.
- *What do they DO?*: this quadrant captures the user's actions and behaviors, such as how they interact with products or services. It helps teams understand the user's habits and routines.
- *What do they HEAR?*: this quadrant captures the user's thoughts and beliefs, such as their goals, motivations, and fears. It helps teams understand the user's mindset and perspective.
- *What do they THINK and FEEL?*: This quadrant captures what thoughts and feelings might motivate user's behavior.
- PAINS: This quadrant captures the user's fears, frustrations, and anxieties are.
- GAINS: This quadrant captures what user's needs, hopes, wants, and dreams are.

Teams then fill in each quadrant with specific details about the user's experience. For example, in the *What the user says* quadrant, they might write down quotes from interviews or customer service calls. In the *What the user does* quadrant, they might sketch out a diagram of the user's workflow or journey through a product or service.

Once the empathy map is complete, teams can use it to identify opportunities for improvement or innovation. For example, they might notice that users frequently express frustration with a particular feature or that they have unmet needs related to a certain aspect of their experience. This information can then be used to inform the design of new products or services that better meet the needs of users.

5.2 Tools and Techniques for Defining the Problem

Understanding the actual issues customers are facing is crucial. Many problems are mentioned by the users during the empathize stage, but the choice of the correct problem that advances the design-thinking process is crucial to its success. Through problem definition, the design team can pinpoint the issue's underlying cause and formulate a clear plan of action. As a result, the design process is more focused and the needs of the user are met by the final solution. A poorly defined problem could lead to the design team wasting time and money on solutions that don't work or don't address the user's needs. Therefore, some of the tools and techniques are used by design teams to determine the correct problem of the users.

5.2.1 Problem Statement

As discussed in the previous chapter, the define stage is related to defining the problem clearly. A problem statement is a clear and concise description of a specific issue or challenge that needs to be addressed. It could benefit greatly from identifying the gap between the current situation and the desired outcome and providing a basis for developing solutions or strategies to solve the problem. Here is an example of a problem statement related to a pizza delivery service:

Problem Statement: The pizza delivery service has low customer retention and satisfaction rates due to late deliveries, inaccurate order tracking, and inconsistent pizza quality. As a result, the service is missing out on potential revenue and failing to build a loyal customer base. To increase customer satisfaction and retention rates, the service must improve its delivery process, improve its tracking system, and ensure consistent quality.

5.2.2 Point-Of-View Statements

Point-of-view statements are used to express a specific viewpoint or position on a given issue or topic. They are frequently used in problem-solving and decision-making processes to help clarify competing viewpoints and guide discussions towards a common understanding. Examples of point-of-view statements include:

- From the customer's perspective, delivery time is the most important factor in choosing a pizza delivery service.
- As a delivery driver, accurate and timely communication with customers is essential to ensuring a positive experience.
- As a pizza chain, prioritizing food safety and quality control in the delivery process to maintain customer trust and loyalty is essential.

- From a business standpoint, offering delivery services can increase revenue and expand the customer base.

Point-of-view statements can be used to facilitate productive discussions and help teams reach a consensus on potential solutions or actions. They can also be used to identify areas of disagreement or conflicting priorities that may need to be addressed before moving forward.

5.2.3 User Needs and Insights

Design-thinking involves understanding the needs and insights of users to define problem that need to be solved. According to Gibbons, S (2019), user need statements, also often called problem statements or point-of-view statements, are the primary tool in the second stage of Design-thinking—the define stage; they align different points of view before moving forward to ideating. Here are some examples of user needs that can help define a problem:

- Consumers want products and services with user-friendly interfaces, clear instructions, and ease of use. For example, customers want quick delivery times and an easy-to-use pizza delivery service.
- Customers want high-quality products and services that are reasonably priced, provide good value, and are of good quality. For example, customers desire a large selection of pizza options, such as gluten-free and vegetarian selections.
- Consumers want products and services that are adaptable to their unique requirements and tastes. For example, users want high-quality ingredients and consistent quality across different locations and franchises.
- Customers want products and services that offer dependable customer service with prompt response times and beneficial guidance. For example, customers want to know that their brand loyalty is valued and rewarded.

Users, even if they claim to, do not always know what they require. According to a well-known quote attributed to Henry Ford, "If I had asked people what they wanted, they would have said faster horses." It is the responsibility of the design team to understand the true needs of their users. Therefore, user insight plays an important role in understanding the real needs of the users. Here is an example of user insight separate from the user's needs.

- Many users have hectic schedules and do not have time to cook, so ordering pizza online is a popular option.
- Some users are concerned about their health and prefer healthier menu options.

- Some customers are concerned about the environmental impact of packaging waste and prefer environmentally friendly packaging options.
- Users frequently rely on social media reviews and recommendations when selecting a pizza delivery service.

5.3 Tools and Techniques for Generating Ideas

The design team will start working on ideas after the problem is defined. Many solutions to the problem may be suggested, however, the decision of which idea to prototype is crucial.Thus, the design team employs a broad range of tools and techniques to identify the idea that best addresses the client's issue. Some such tools and techniques are discussed below:

5.3.1 Brainstorming

Brainstorming is a well-known technique for generating ideas in a group setting. Design thinkers come up with as many ideas as possible without judgment, encouraging creativity and collaboration. Brainstorming aims to generate as many ideas as possible, without judgment or criticism. The focus is on quantity, not quality, and the goal is to generate a broad range of ideas that can be refined and narrowed down later in the design process.

During a brainstorming session, participants are encouraged to build on each other's ideas, think outside the box, and avoid self-censorship. Ideas are captured on sticky notes or whiteboards, and there is no hierarchy or ranking of ideas.

Once the brainstorming session is complete, the ideas are reviewed and evaluated based on their potential impact, feasibility, and alignment with the project goals. The most promising ideas are selected for further development and refinement, while less promising ideas are set aside.

Brainstorming is a powerful tool for generating innovative solutions to complex problems. It encourages creativity, collaboration, and open-mindedness, and it can lead to breakthrough insights and ideas that might not have been possible through individual thinking alone (Müller-Roterberg, 2020).

5.3.2 Selecting Ideas

- **Dot-voting:** is a technique used in group settings to prioritize or vote on ideas or options. Each person is given a set number of dots (usually stickers or markers), which they place next to the ideas or options they most strongly support. The concept or option with the most dots is declared the winner. In brainstorming sessions, team meetings, and decision-making processes, dot-voting is frequently used. It is a quick and easy way to gather feedback and reach a consensus.

- **Thumb Method:** is a quick and easy way to get feedback or opinions from a group of people. This is how it works:
  - Ask the group a question or make a statement.
  - Have everyone hold up their thumb in one of three different positions:
    - *Up:* if they agree with the statement or question.
    - *Sideways:* if they are undecided or neutral.
    - *Down:* if they disagree with the statement or question.
  - To get an idea of the group's overall opinion, count the number of thumbs in each position.

  The Thumb Method is frequently used in meetings, workshops, and other group settings that require quick feedback. Facilitators can use it to gauge the group's level of agreement or disagreement on a particular idea.
- **Five-Finger Method:** This method is also widely used for getting quick feedback. Everyone needs to show number of fingers as below:
  - **Five fingers:** the idea is great.
  - **Four fingers:** the idea is good.
  - **Three fingers:** the idea is interesting.
  - **Two fingers:** the idea has weaknesses.
  - **One finger:** the idea should be rejected.
- **Card Sequence:** write the idea on a card or sticky note in keywords. After a discussion among team members, sort the cards or notes from left (very good idea) - to right (poor idea). Ideas with the same rating are positioned on top of each other.

5.3.3 Mind Mapping

As discussed in Chapter 3 mind mapping can be a great tool for idea selection because it allows design teams to visually organize and connect their ideas. Here are some steps that can be taken to use mind mapping for idea selection:

- Start by writing down the main topic or problem in the center of a blank page.
- Begin brainstorming ideas related to the topic or problem, writing each idea on a separate branch connected to the center.

- As more ideas are generated, start to group them into categories or themes. Use different colors or shapes to distinguish between different categories.
- Evaluate each idea based on its potential impact and feasibility, similar to the Card Sequence Method.
- Prioritize the ideas based on their impact and feasibility and use the mind map to identify connections and relationships between ideas.
- Test and refine the selected ideas, similar to the Card Sequence Method.

By using mind mapping for idea selection, design thinkers can create a visual representation of their ideas that makes it easier to see connections and identify promising ideas.

5.3.4 SWOT Analysis

SWOT analysis is a strategic planning tool used to identify and analyze the strengths, weaknesses, opportunities, and threats of a product, service, or organization. It involves examining both internal and external factors that can impact the success of a project or business, as shown in Figure 5.5.

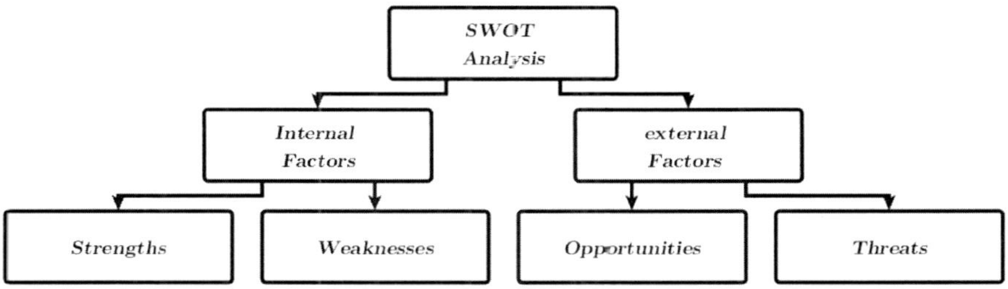

Figure 5.5: SWOT Analysis

- **Strengths:** are the internal factors that give a product or service an edge over rivals. This could involve unique attributes, a well-known brand, or an accomplished group of employees.
- **Weaknesses:** are the internal factors that make a product or service less advantageous than rivals. Examples of this could be inadequate resources, outdated technology, or poor client service.
- **Opportunities:** are external factors that can be used to increase a product or service's chances of success. This could involve shifting consumer behavior, new market trends, or developing technologies.
- **Threats:** are external factors that have the potential to harm a product or service's success. This can involve shifts in regulations, the entry of new rivals into the market, or economic downturns.

Consider the SWOT analysis of a tracking system that allows people to track pizza orders in real time. Here is how a SWOT analysis could be performed for this idea, as shown in Figure 5.6:

Strengths: *- Gives customers more control over their delivery experience by tracking pizza orders in real-time;* *- Can boost customer satisfaction by lowering wait times and uncertainty;* *- Can assist the business in streamlining delivery routes and increasing efficiency;* *- Can offer useful information on customer preferences and behaviors*	*Weakness:* *- May not be cost-effective for smaller pizza companies;* *- Dependency on third-party delivery services may limit control over the delivery process;* *- May not be effective in areas with poor GPS or internet connectivity;* *- Requires significant investment in technology and infrastructure to implement.*
Opportunities: *- Stand out from competitors by providing a one-of-a-kind and innovative service.* *- Extend the tracking system to include additional food delivery or service options.* *- Collaborate with popular food delivery apps to reach a larger audience.* *- Use tracking system data to inform marketing and advertising efforts.*	*Threats:* *- Competitors may create similar tracking systems, reducing the service's novelty.* *- Negative reviews or technical problems with the tracking system may harm the company's reputation.* *- Customers may not see the value in the tracking system and prefer traditional delivery methods.* *- Concerns about privacy may arise in connection with the collection and use of customer data.*

Figure 5.6: Tracking System Using SWOT Analysis

By conducting a SWOT analysis, design thinkers can gain a better understanding of the current state of their product or service and identify areas for improvement. This can help inform the design process and ensure that the final product meets the needs of both the business and its customers.

5.3.5 Sketching

The process of ideation sketching involves visualizing concepts and ideas to investigate and refine them. The process entails producing brief, rough sketches that distill a notion or idea without becoming bogged down in specifics. A variety of tools, such as pen and paper, whiteboards, or digital sketching software, can be used for ideation sketching. The objective is to generate a variety of ideas and investigate various possibilities, rather than produce a polished or finished product.

According to Rojas, J. (2023), it is a common misconception that the purpose of sketches in the design process is the same as that of low-fidelity prototyping, but this is not true. Table 5.2 shows the differences between sketches and prototypes.

Table 5.2: Sketches vs Prototypes

Sketches	Prototypes
Sketches are quick, informal drawings used to experiment with and communicate ideas.	Prototypes are more detailed than sketches but less refined.
Sketches are typically created on paper or digitally and can be easily modified or discarded as new ideas emerge.	Prototypes are physical or digital representations of a design that are tested and evaluated for basic functionality and usability.
Sketches are not highly detailed or refined.	Prototypes are typically made of low-cost materials and can be quickly iterated upon as feedback is received.
Sketches are typically used during the ideation phase of the design process when the goal is to generate as many ideas as possible.	Prototypes are used in the prototyping phase of the design process, where the emphasis is on testing and refining a design.

Teams can collaborate to develop and refine their ideas by sketching them out, resulting in stronger and more innovative solutions. Sketches are quick, informal drawings used for ideation, whereas low-fidelity prototypes are more detailed representations used for testing and refining a design.

5.4 Prototyping

Once an idea is formed, it moves to a prototype for testing. As discussed in the previous chapter, prototypes can be divided into two types: low-fidelity prototypes and high-fidelity prototypes. Dam, R.F. and Teo, Y.S. (2016), proposed five well-known prototyping tools as below:

5.4.1 Sketching

Sketching can be used at nearly any stage in the product design process; drawing out brainstormed ideas, recording every "aha" moments, or building prototypes. The 'aha' moment is one of sudden insight or discovery. Prototyping is a way to give design ideas a presence so that design thinkers can test them out or put them in front of people to see if they have value (Cui, S., 2018). Sketches are very useful for decision-making, even though they are frequently regarded as not technically prototypes. This is primarily because they are very simple to make and even simpler to discard. This is an excellent tool for both design thinkers and non-design thinkers because drawing well doesn't require artistic talent. The advantages and disadvantages of sketching are shown in Table 5.3.

Table 5.3: Advantages and Disadvantages of Sketching

Advantages	Disadvantages
Sketches can be made quickly and for a very low cost. As a result, an extensive number of ideas can be produced quickly.	Sketches lack detail and are intentionally ambiguous. As a result, they cannot be used to convey complex interactions
Sketches can be completed anywhere using a pen and paper or digitally on a desktop, tablet, or smartphone.	Sketches are rarely of sufficient fidelity to be useful with people outside the team because they rarely have the context to understand what the sketch is trying to convey.
Sketching improves the artist's observation skills by requiring them to focus on details and nuances in the subject they are drawing.	Other types of prototypes, like paper prototypes or wireframes, are more useful in convergent processes where design thinkers typically choose the few best ideas. Sketches are not very helpful in these situations.

5.4.2 Paper Prototypes

For more interactive testing and evaluation of the design, a paper prototype is usually preferred over a sketch. A paper prototype is a physical representation of the design that users can work with and test to find any problems with usability or errors in the design.

Interactivity is the main distinction between simple sketches and a paper prototype. A member of the design team breathes life into a paper prototype by rearranging components, creating unique responses, and sometimes vocally announcing certain effects that are too difficult to depict on paper. This simulates what computer would do in response to the user's *clicks* and *keystrokes*. Design thinkers can user-test a paper prototype by assigning users a task and observing how they complete it since it is interactive. It is evident that a paper prototype has low fidelity in terms of appearance and feel. However, it can achieve high fidelity in terms of breadth, covering a wide range of features or functionality, all at a very minimal cost (Snyder, 2003).

Paper prototypes are often used in the early stages of the design process to test different design options and get feedback from users. They are quick and inexpensive to create, making them an ideal tool for rapid prototyping and iteration.

While sketches can be useful for visualizing ideas and exploring different design options, they are not as effective at simulating the user experience or identifying usability issues. On the other hand, paper prototypes provide a more realistic representation of the design and allow users to interact with it more meaningfully. The advantages and disadvantages of a paper prototype are shown in Table 5.4.

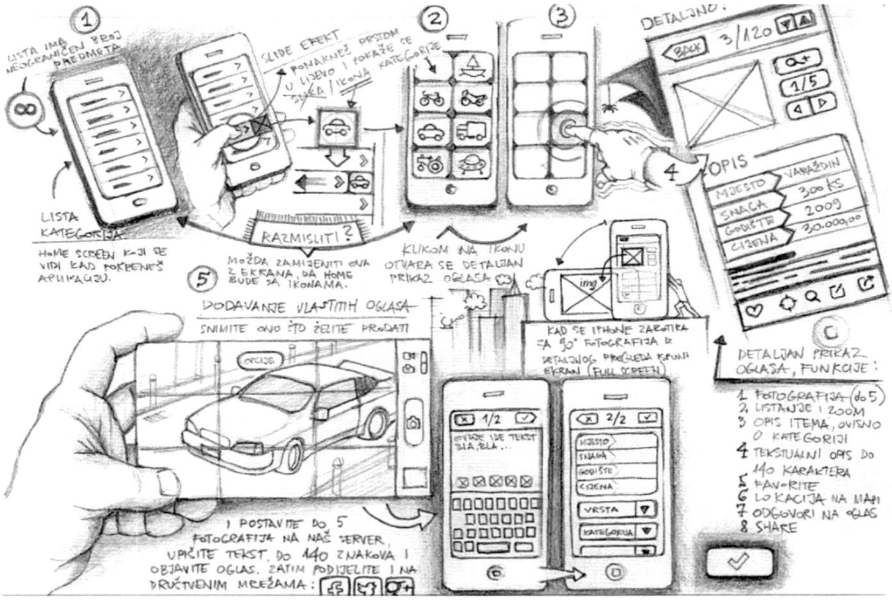

Figure 5.7: Paper Prototype Example(Source: Cui, S. (2018))

Table 5.4: Advantages and Disadvantages of Paper Prototypes

Advantages	**Disadvantages**
Prototypes made of paper can be easily and affordably created and modified.	Although generally simple to construct, creating a paper prototype may occasionally take some time, and sometimes it can be difficult to make bigger, more structural changes.
It can use sliding pieces of paper to create crude *animations* that give users a more realistic preview of how the interface will function.	Paper prototypes are less useful for testing UI patterns that are frequently used. This is because users probably already understand how the UI functions.
It can overlook the subtler, more surface-level aspects of an interface, like a button's color. This makes it possible for design thinkers to test the idea itself, rather than just how it looks.	Paper prototypes can only be tested in person. It will be quite difficult to perform remote tests with the physical prototype.
Users are unlikely to withhold their criticism of paper prototypes out of concern that they will offend someone because they are unfinished.	Paper prototypes are an improvement over sketches, however, users still need to use their imagination. This implies that some users may find it difficult to comprehend how the interface functions.

5.4.3 Lego Prototypes

A Lego prototype is an actual model made with Lego bricks that demonstrates a design. It is a widely used prototyping technique in fields like engineering, architecture, and product design. Lego prototypes are frequently used to build 3D models of designs, giving designers a tangible means of testing and visualizing their concepts. LEGO's versatility allows for the quick and easy creation of prototypes, enabling rapid prototyping. They are quick and simple to assemble, disassemble, and adjust. Prototyping companies have started experimenting with combining 3D printing—which is slow to build—with LEGO pieces to create physical prototypes more quickly. This allows 3D printing to be restricted to the portion of the physical prototype that is being tested. The benefits of using LEGO prototypes are as follows:

- LEGO prototypes can produce physical models much more quickly than most 3D printers.
- LEGO prototypes are simple to put together and take apart, which makes it easy to tweak and refine the design.
- LEGO prototypes are accessible to design thinkers of all stripes because they are reasonably priced for producing physical, tangible, and widely available product prototypes.
- LEGO prototypes are adaptable and simple to alter, which is helpful during the product development process's exploratory phases.

Although Lego prototypes are an enjoyable and practical approach to testing and exploring designs, they have some weaknesses which are explained below:

- Digital products like websites and mobile apps shouldn't use Lego prototypes. They can still be utilized, nevertheless, to write user journey narratives for these intangible goods.
- Low-fidelity Lego prototypes can be costly, particularly if designers have to purchase a set of Lego bricks which are more expensive than paper prototypes or other types of prototypes.

5.4.4 Digital Wireframes

A wireframe is a basic, bare-bones illustration of an application or website. It enables the focus to be on the functionality and content organization rather than the interactive and visual elements of the prototype. Low-fidelity wireframes are what paper prototypes are technically referred to. Visual representations of the design and functionality of a website or application are called digital wireframes. Usually composed of basic design elements such as text and simple shapes, they are produced through the use of specialized software or tools. The structure and content of a digital product, including where buttons, menus, and other interactive elements are placed, are communicated through wireframes. Before beginning more in-depth design work, they aid stakeholders and design thinkers in visualizing and improving the user experience, which makes them a crucial component of the design process. The use of wireframes gives a wide variety of benefits, as below:

- Wireframes, as opposed to higher-fidelity prototypes such as app mockups, can be changed quickly. This is because wireframes lack details such as images and colors.
- Wireframes concentrate on the functionality and content structure of the product. Furthermore, rather than visual preferences, users will direct their feedback toward functional issues.
- When compared to other low-fidelity prototypes, wireframes communicate the relationship between different product pages. Users and team members can easily see where each page leads and what each button does.

While wireframing has many advantages, there are a few drawbacks that should not be disregarded. These are some significant disadvantages:

- Wireframes lack the detail found in high-fidelity designs, making it difficult to visualize the finished product.
- Wireframes only provide a basic representation of the functionality of a website or application, making it difficult to test specific features.
- Wireframes are frequently simple and lack the visual appeal of high-fidelity designs.
- Wireframes are not always appropriate for projects that require a strong emphasis on visual design or complex functionality.

5.4.5 Wizard of Oz

A Wizard of Oz prototype entails developing a simulated version of a product or service that appears fully functional but is controlled by a human *wizard* behind the scenes. This type of prototype is used to test the user experience of a product or service without having to build it. The name *Wizard of Oz* is derived from the famous scene in the book and film in which the wizard is revealed to be an ordinary man behind a curtain operating a machine. The advantages and disadvantages of Wizard of Oz are shown in Table 5.5.

5.5 Tools and Techniques Used for Testing

Design-thinking requires testing because it allows design thinkers to test and validate their ideas with users. Design-thinking is a user-centered

Table 5.5: Advantages and Disadvantages of Wizard of Oz

Advantages	Disadvantages
It is used to test particularly complex parts of a design without having to build it. This allows validation of the design before investing more resources in its implementation.	Takes time to build the Wizard of Oz prototype because it must persuade the user that it is fully functional, and it must appear convincingly polished.
Also used to test future technologies without having to build a complicated prototype. This allows fine-tuning the technology's requirements.	Must train a *wizard* who will simulate the system's responses. The wizard must also be present during all tests, which takes more time and effort.
Users are more likely to provide realistic feedback because Wizard of Oz prototypes are more believable and interactive.	The wizard may not behave consistently throughout the tests. As a result, the system may behave differently from test to test, influencing the results. This means special attention to training wizards and establishing ground rules for them to follow is impertive.

problem-solving approach that includes understanding users' needs and preferences, developing solutions, prototyping them, and testing them. Testing is an important step in the Design-thinking process because it allows design thinkers to get feedback on their prototypes, identify areas for improvement, and refine their ideas.

Designers can conduct structured and systematic user testing. Tools can assist design thinkers in creating and distributing surveys, conducting interviews, gathering feedback, and analyzing data. Design thinkers can collect quantitative and qualitative data about how users interact with their prototypes by using testing tools. This information can be used to make educated decisions about how to enhance the user experience and refine the design.

Design thinkers can also use testing tools to iterate quickly. They can identify problems and make improvements by testing early and frequently before investing too much time and resources in a particular solution. This assists design thinkers in developing more comprehensive products that meet the needs of users. Overall, testing tools are an important part of the design-thinking process, assisting design thinkers in developing effective and meaningful user-centered solutions.

5.5.1 User Testing

Observing and collecting feedback from users as they interact with prototypes helps design thinkers identify flaws, validate assumptions, and make necessary improvements. User testing is a crucial part of the design-thinking process that involves gathering feedback from actual users on a prototype or product. The goal of user testing is to identify any usability issues, gather insights on user behavior and preferences, and refine the design to better meet the needs of users.

User testing typically involves recruiting a group of users who represent the target audience for the product or service. These users are then given a set of tasks to perform using the prototype or product, while a moderator observes and records their behavior and feedback.

During user testing, design thinkers may use a variety of methods to gather feedback, including surveys, interviews, observation, and usability testing. Usability testing involves asking users to complete specific tasks using the prototype or product while the designer observes and records any issues or challenges they encounter.

Once user testing is complete, design thinkers analyze the feedback and make changes to the prototype or product based on the insights gathered. This iterative process continues until the design meets the needs of users and aligns with project goals.

User testing is a critical component of the design-thinking process because it ensures that the final product or service meets the needs of users and provides a positive user experience. By gathering feedback early in the design process, design thinkers can make changes that lead to a more comprehensive final product, ultimately increasing user satisfaction and adoption. According to Torsten, T. (2019), there are two main types of user testing:

- Moderated User Test
- Unmoderated User Test

5.5.1.1 Moderated User Test

Moderated user testing happens when a user performs particular tasks on a product or service while being observed in real time by a researcher. During a moderated user test, design teams can guide test users through tasks, probe and dig deeper into problems, and receive real-time feedback. The benefit of moderated user testing is that it allows users to investigate problems in real-time, but the drawbacks are biases and facilitation. Advantages of moderated user testing are:

- Allows for more in-depth feedback and observation of the user's behavior.
- Provides an opportunity to ask follow-up questions and clarify any confusion.
- Allows for real-time adjustments to the testing process based on the user's behavior and feedback.

Although Moderated user testing provides several benefits, it also has some disadvantages. The disadvantages of moderated user testing include:

- Can be more time-consuming and expensive than unmoderated testing.
- May introduce bias if the moderator inadvertently influences the user's behavior or feedback.
- It requires scheduling and coordinating with participants and the moderator.

5.5.1.2 Unmoderated User Test

Unmoderated user testing, on the other hand, is done remotely without the presence of a moderator. Users are assigned tasks to complete on their own, and their interactions with the prototype are documented. This type of testing is frequently carried out via online platforms that enable remote testing and data collection. Unmoderated testing is generally less expensive and faster than moderated testing, but it may not provide as much insight into user thought processes or behaviors. Advantages and disadvantages of unmoderated user testing can be seen in Table 5.6.

Table 5.6: Advantage vs Disadvantages of Unmoderated User Testing

Advantages	Disadvantages
Can be faster and less expensive than moderated testing.	May not provide as much insight into the user's thought process or behavior.
Allows for a larger sample size since participants can complete the tasks conveniently.	It is difficult to ask follow-up questions or clarify any confusion during the testing process.
Reduces the potential for bias since no moderator is present to influence the user's behavior or feedback.	Requires careful planning and design to ensure the tasks are clear and easy to understand.

5.5.2 Usability Testing

Usability testing is a technique for evaluating the user experience of a product or service by observing how users interact with it. The purpose of usability testing is to identify any usability issues or barriers that may prevent users from completing tasks or achieving their goals, as well as to make recommendations for improving the user experience. Types of usability testing include the following:

- **Moderated Usability Testing:** a facilitator introduces the test to participants, answers their queries, and asks follow-up questions
- **Unmoderated Usability Testing:** participants conduct the test without direct supervision, usually with a script.
- **Remote Usability Testing:** test participants (and the researcher, in the case of moderated usability testing) conduct the test online or, more rarely, over the phone.

- **In-Person Usability Testing:** test participants and the researcher(s) are in the same location.

Although usability and user testing are sometimes used synonymously, their purposes are not the same (Hotjar, 2023). User testing is a research method that uses real people to evaluate a product or service by observing their interactions and gathering feedback. Compared to usability testing, insights from user testing reveal:

- What users think about when using a product or service.
- How they perceive the product or service.
- What are the relevant user needs?

Usability testing, on the other hand, has a more focused approach, by seeking to answer questions like:

- Are there bugs or other errors impacting user flow?
- Can users complete their tasks efficiently?
- Do they understand how to navigate the site?

5.5.2.1 Why is Usability Testing Important?

Real-world users test products for usability, and they are likely to find problems that experts in the field miss. Design thinkers, marketers, and product owners frequently overlook usability problems in their products because of their extensive knowledge. Usability testing is important for several reasons:

1. Usability testing aids in the identification of any usability concerns or issues that users might run into when utilizing a service or product. This data can be utilized to enhance the product's functionality and design.
2. Usability testing assists in enhancing the user experience by pinpointing potential trouble spots or points of frustration for users. The product can be made easier to use and more user-friendly by fixing these problems.
3. Usability testing can help identify issues early in the development process, saving time and money in the long run. Developers can save money on redesigns by addressing usability issues early on.
4. Usability testing improves customer satisfaction, implying that a product that is simple to use and understand is more likely to please customers. Usability testing ensures that a product meets the needs and expectations of its users.
5. Usability testing provides a competitive advantage by improving the usability of a product. Customers are more likely to prefer a product that is easy to use and understand than a similar product with poor usability.

All things considered, usability testing is crucial because it guarantees that a product is easy to use, fulfills user needs, and is competitive in the market.

5.5.3 A/B Testing

In A/B testing, two iterations of a product, website, application, or concept are compared to see which works better. It is a methodical approach to determining the optimal version of the work. A/B testing, sometimes referred to as split testing or bucket testing, is essentially an experiment in which users are randomly shown two options. Afterward, statistical analysis is used by analysts, developers, marketers, and design thinkers to ascertain which variation best meets their desired results. The goal of A/B testing is to determine the user's preference.

5.5.3.1 What Are the Benefits of A/B Testing?

According to Bruton, L. (2022), in many fields, including marketing, data analytics, user experience (UX) and user interface (UI), A/B testing eliminates the need for conjecture. Design professionals can make sure they are truly producing a strong outcome by using A/B testing to measure the impact of any changes they make. By testing their designs, design thinkers can enhance their products and ensure that they satisfy customer needs. Another advantage of A/B testing for businesses is long-term cost savings, especially when it is done in the design phase. Testing often finds mistakes or subpar designs before development.

5.5.3.2 Why is A/B Testing Important?

A/B testing is an important technique used to improve the performance of a product or service. Here are some reasons why A/B testing is important:

- A/B testing can be used to settle a design team conflict, as it provides objective data that can help resolve disagreements and guide decision-making. By testing different versions of a design, the team can evaluate which approach is more effective based on metrics such as engagement, conversion rates, and user feedback. This data can then be used to inform further iterations and improvements to the design.
- A/B testing is a method of comparing two versions of a design to determine which one performs better. It involves randomly assigning users to one of two groups, with each group seeing a different version of the design. By tracking user behavior and engagement, such as click-through rates, conversion rates, or time spent on a page, design thinkers can gather quantitative data about the effectiveness of each version.
- A/B testing can help design thinkers make informed decisions that are focused on the needs and preferences of users. By testing two different versions of a design with real users, design thinkers can gather data on how users interact with each version and which one is more effective in achieving the desired outcome.

- A/B testing can help confirm the validity of a design change. If the A/B test shows that the design change has a positive impact on user behavior or achieves the desired outcome, then it can be concluded that the design change is valid. On the other hand, if the A/B test shows that the design change does not have a positive impact or even harms user behavior, then it can be concluded that the design change is not valid and will not benefit implementation.

5.5.4 Accessibility Testing

The process of design-thinking includes accessibility testing as a crucial step. Testing a design to make sure it is usable by everyone, including people with impairments, is part of it. Examining a product or service for accessibility can assist design thinkers in identifying any possible obstacles that might keep some users from using or accessing it.

As part of the design-thinking process, accessibility testing usually entails conducting user testing with people who have various disabilities, such as hearing, vision, or mobility impairments. The purpose of this testing is to find any problems or difficulties that these users might run into while utilizing the good or service.

It is possible to test accessibility manually or automatically. Some common accessibility problems, like inadequate color contrast, missing alt text for images, and keyboard accessibility, can be found with the aid of automated tools. But not all accessibility issues—like how well-structured the content is, how understandable the instructions are, or how well the website or app functions with assistive technologies—can be found by automated tools.

Consequently, manual testing is also required to verify that the website or app is functional and easy to use from the viewpoint of various users with varying needs and preferences. In manual testing, real users with disabilities or impairments can be used as test subjects, as well as accessibility checklists and assistive technologies like screen readers and speech recognition software.

Design thinkers can produce products and services that are more inclusive and accessible to all users, regardless of their abilities or disabilities, by integrating accessibility testing into the design-thinking process. This promotes diversity and social inclusion in addition to making the user experience better for all users.

5.5.5 Performance Testing

Performance testing can be extremely useful in the design-thinking process because it allows designers to evaluate the effectiveness of their solutions. Performance testing assesses a product or system's speed, responsiveness, and stability under various conditions. It enables designers to identify and address any performance issues that may affect the user experience. It entails evaluating the performance of a product or service under various conditions to ensure that it meets the desired performance criteria. In design-thinking, performance testing can be used to:

1. **Verify Hypotheses:** design thinkers can verify their predictions about how a product or service will function in the real world by putting it to the test and seeing how it performs. This can assist them in spotting possible problems and making the required adjustments before the product or service's launch.
2. **Design Optimization:** by pinpointing areas in which changes can be made, performance testing assists designers in making their designs more effective. For instance, when a website loads slowly, performance testing can assist designers in determining the root cause and implementing the required adjustments to speed up the process.
3. **Assess Success:** another method for assessing a product or service's success is performance testing. Design thinkers can monitor progress and make necessary adjustments to ensure that the product or service is meeting its objectives by establishing performance benchmarks.

All things considered, performance testing is a crucial step in the Design-thinking process because it aids in the development of practical and efficient solutions.

5.6 Review Advanced Design-Thinking Tools

Design-thinking is crucial for future designers because it provides a structured approach to problem-solving that is centered around the needs and experiences of users. By incorporating empathy, experimentation, and iteration into the design process, design thinkers can create solutions that are not only innovative but also effective and user-friendly. Design-thinking also encourages collaboration and cross-functional teamwork, which is essential in today's complex and rapidly changing business environment. Additionally, as technology continues to evolve, design thinkers who are skilled in data analysis and the use of virtual and augmented reality tools will be in high demand. Finally, with a growing focus on sustainability and ethical considerations, design thinkers who can integrate these principles into their work will be well-positioned for success in the future.

5.6.1 Virtual Reality (VR) and Augmented Reality (AR) Tools

Virtual Reality (VR) and Augmented Reality (AR) tools can help designers create immersive experiences for users, allowing them to test and refine their designs in a virtual environment. Dehant, B. (2023), mentioned that VR has the potential to be an important tool for design-thinking, offering a distinctive and immersive way to comprehend users' demands, produce and test design ideas, and develop useful solutions. These tools are becoming increasingly popular in the design-thinking process.

VR tools allow designers to create a completely digital environment that users can interact with. This can be useful for testing out designs for products or environments that do not yet exist, such as a new car or a building. By creating a virtual environment, design thinkers can test out different design ideas and see how they work in practice before investing in expensive physical prototypes.

AR tools, on the other hand, allow design thinkers to overlay digital elements in the real world. This can be useful for testing out designs for products that will be used in the real world, such as a new piece of furniture or a smartphone app. By overlaying digital elements in the real world, design thinkers can see how their designs will look and feel in context, allowing them to make adjustments as needed. Some examples of VR and AR tools are as follows:

5.6.1.1 Sketchbox

One example of a VR tool is Sketchbox[1]. Sketchbox is a virtual reality design tool that allows teams to create and test prototypes in a 3D environment. It is essentially a virtual workspace that provides a range of tools and features for artists and design thinkers to create, edit, and refine their virtual creations.

Users can use hand-held controllers or other input devices to interact with the Sketchbox, which appears as a 3D environment within VR headset. They can draw, sculpt, paint, and manipulate objects in real time, using a variety of brushes, textures, and materials. Sketchbox also includes features such as lighting, shading, and camera controls, which allow users to experiment with different visual effects and perspectives.

One of the main advantages of Sketchbox in VR is the ability to provide a more immersive and intuitive creative experience. Allowing users to work in a virtual space that closely resembles the real world, can help to break down some of the barriers that exist between the artist's vision and the final product. Additionally, Sketchbox can be used collaboratively, allowing multiple users to work on the same project simultaneously from different locations. With Sketchbox, teams can quickly iterate on designs and get feedback from users in a more immersive way than traditional prototyping methods.

---

[1] `https://design.sketchbox3d.com/`

5.6.1.2 Gravity Sketch

Another example of a VR tool is Gravity Sketch. Gravity Sketch is a 3D design tool that allows teams to create and manipulate 3D models in virtual reality. It is similar to Sketchbox VR, but with some unique features and capabilities.

Users can use hand-held controllers or other input devices to interact with Gravity Sketch, which appears as a 3D environment within the VR headset. They can draw, sculpt, paint, and manipulate objects in real-time, using a variety of brushes, textures, and materials. Gravity Sketch also includes features such as symmetry tools, mirroring, and snapping, which allow users to create precise and symmetrical designs.

One of the main advantages of Gravity Sketch VR is its ability to provide a more intuitive and natural creative experience. Allowing users to work in a virtual space that closely resembles the real world, can help to break down some of the barriers that exist between the artist's vision and the final product. Additionally, Gravity Sketch in VR can be used collaboratively, allowing multiple users to work on the same project simultaneously from different locations.

Gravity Sketch has been widely adopted by design thinkers, architects, and engineers for its ability to quickly prototype and iterate on complex 3D designs. It has also been used in industries such as automotive design, product design, and virtual reality game development. With Gravity Sketch, teams can quickly prototype and test new product designs, and get feedback from users in real-time.

5.6.1.3 ARKit

ARKit is a software development kit created by Apple that allows developers to create augmented reality (AR) experiences for iOS devices. ARKit uses the device's camera and sensors to detect the environment and place virtual objects within it, creating an immersive and interactive experience.

ARKit includes features such as motion tracking, which allows virtual objects to move and interact with the real world in real time, and environmental understanding, which enables the device to recognize and respond to the physical environment. It also includes advanced rendering techniques such as lighting estimation, which allows virtual objects to appear more realistic by adapting to the lighting conditions of the environment.

ARKit has been widely adopted by developers for a variety of applications, including gaming, education, retail, and entertainment. It has also been used in industries such as architecture, interior design, and product visualization, allowing users to preview and interact with virtual designs in real-world settings.

5.6.1.4 ARCore

ARCore is a software development kit created by Google that allows developers to create augmented reality (AR) experiences for Android devices. ARCore uses the device's camera and sensors to detect the environment and place virtual objects within it, creating an immersive and interactive experience.

ARCore includes features such as motion tracking, which allows virtual objects to move and interact with the real world in real time, and environmental understanding, which enables the device to recognize and respond to the physical environment. It also includes advanced rendering techniques such as lighting estimation, which allows virtual objects to appear more realistic by adapting to the lighting conditions of the environment.

ARCore has been widely adopted by developers for a variety of applications, including gaming, education, retail, and entertainment. It has also been used in industries such as architecture, interior design, and product visualization, allowing users to preview and interact with virtual designs in real-world settings.

Overall, VR and AR tools are powerful tools in Design-thinking as they allow teams to create more immersive and interactive experiences that can help them better understand user needs and behaviors. By leveraging these tools, teams can create more innovative and user-centered products and services.

5.6.2 Artificial Intelligence (AI) Tools

Artificial Intelligence (AI) Tools can be used to analyze user data and behavior, providing design thinkers with insights into how users interact with their products and services. These tools are becoming increasingly popular in the design-thinking process. These tools use machine learning algorithms to analyze data and provide insights that can inform the design process.

5.6.2.1 Predictive Analytics

Predictive analytics, which uses data to forecast future trends and behaviors, is an AI tool used in design-thinking. With this information, designers can make products that have a higher chance of succeeding in the marketplace. AI tools for design-thinking feature predictive analytics, which is a technology that analyzes data and forecasts future results using machine learning algorithms. This tool can assist developers and design thinkers in understanding user behavior and preferences, spotting possible issues or opportunities, and projecting future trends.

Predictive analytics, for instance, can be used to examine user data and spot trends in user behavior, such as the most often-used features of a product or the most popular sections of a website. The design process can then be informed by this data, enabling designers to produce products that more effectively satisfy the requirements and preferences of their target audience.

Predictive analytics can also be used to spot possible issues or opportunities and forecast future trends. For instance, design thinkers can spot new trends and create products that have a higher chance of becoming well-liked down the road by examining social media data and search trends. In a similar vein, design thinkers can spot possible flaws in a product and address them before they become serious problems by examining user comments and product reviews.

5.6.2.2 Natural Language Processing (NLP)

The technology that allows computers to comprehend, interpret, and produce human language is known as natural language processing, or NLP. NLP is useful in the design-thinking context for processing and analyzing vast amounts of textual data, including social media posts, product reviews, and customer feedback.

NLP, for instance, can be used to examine client feedback and spot recurring themes or problems. The design process can then be informed by this data, enabling designers to produce goods that cater to the wants and needs of their target market.

Natural language responses to user queries can also be produced by NLP, for example, by chatbots or virtual assistants. NLP can enhance user experience and facilitate customer interaction with a product or service by interpreting user input and producing relevant responses.

5.6.2.3 Adobe Sensei

Adobe Sensei is an AI-powered tool that improves the design-thinking process through the use of NLP and machine learning algorithms. It is capable of analyzing vast volumes of text, video, and image data and producing insights that can guide the design process.

Design thinkers can concentrate on more creative aspects of the design process by using Adobe Sensei to automate repetitive tasks like image editing and tagging. Based on user data and behavior, it can also be used to create personalized content, like product recommendations or focused marketing messages.

Adobe Sensei can also be integrated with other Adobe products, like Illustrator, Photoshop, and InDesign, to give designers access to even more sophisticated features and functionalities. For instance, depending on the design's content, it may recommend certain color schemes or typeface selections.

5.6.2.4 Canva's Magic Resize feature

Canva is a graphic design platform that automatically resizes designs to fit various digital channels and social media platforms using artificial intelligence. Because it eliminates the need to manually resize designs for each platform, this feature saves design thinkers time and effort. Design thinkers can quickly and simply resize their designs for various platforms and formats with Canva's AI-powered Magic Resize feature. Design thinkers can use this tool to create a single design and then use the Magic Resize feature to have multiple versions of the design automatically generated in various aspect ratios and sizes.

The Magic Resize feature automatically resizes text, images, and spacing to fit the new dimensions by first analyzing the original design using machine learning algorithms. Design thinkers can now save time and effort by not having to manually resize and modify their designs for every platform or format.

The Magic Resize feature can be used to create variations of a design, like altering the font style or color scheme, in addition to resizing. This makes it easier for designers to rapidly refine their concepts and test various iterations to determine which ones perform the best.

In addition, artificial intelligence (AI) tools can be applied to user research, such as sentiment analysis on social media posts and user behavior analysis on websites and apps. The user experience can then be enhanced by using this data to guide design choices. In conclusion, design thinkers can benefit from AI tools by streamlining their processes, gaining knowledge from user data, and producing more effective and customized designs. AI integration into the Design-thinking process enables teams to produce more inventive and customer-focused goods and services.

5.6.3 Collaboration Tools

The design-thinking process requires collaboration, and collaboration tools are critical to enabling productive teamwork. Collaboration tools are computer programs that let groups and individuals collaborate on projects, talk, and exchange data instantly, no matter where they are in the world. Collaboration tools like video conferencing software and virtual whiteboards will be more and more necessary for design thinkers to collaborate efficiently as remote work becomes more prevalent.

Digital whiteboards are among the tools that enable teams to collaborate on ideas and sketches even when they are not in the same physical space. Teams can improve idea visualization and refinement with the aid of this tool. Furthermore, real-time collaboration on projects, task delegation, and progress tracking is made possible by additional tools such as project management software. Throughout the design-thinking process, this tool can assist teams in remaining structured and on task.

5.6.3.1 Mural

Mural is a collaboration tool used in design-thinking. Regardless of location, teams can work together and generate ideas in real-time using the mural, a digital workspace. It provides a number of tools, including sticky notes, templates, and diagrams, to assist groups in visualizing their concepts and cooperating to produce solutions. Mural provides a variety of design-thinking frameworks and templates, including empathy maps, customer journey maps, and user personas. Teams can work together more productively and organize their ideation process with the aid of these templates.

Additionally, the tool has features like video conferencing, drawing tools, and sticky notes that make it easy for teams to communicate and work together. Teams can easily share and collaborate across platforms by using Mural's integration with other tools like Google Drive, Trello, and Slack. All things considered, Mural is a strong Design-thinking tool that lets teams collaborate virtually and produce excellent designs via efficient ideation and visual cooperation.

5.6.3.2 Figma

With Figma, designers can collaborate in real time on a single project using an interface design tool. Teams can communicate and iterate on designs more effectively with the help of features like version control and commenting. A team can work on the same design at the same time with Figma's collaborative features, which facilitate real-time ideas and feedback sharing. Additionally, interactive prototypes can be made with the tool and shared with stakeholders for testing and feedback.

By ensuring that everyone in the team is working on the most recent version of the design, Figma's version control feature lowers the possibility of mistakes and inconsistencies. Additionally, the tool integrates with other collaboration tools, including Jira, Trello, and Slack, making it simple to share designs and work together across platforms. All things considered, Figma is a strong design-thinking tool that lets teams collaborate virtually and produce excellent digital products via efficient prototyping and collaboration.

5.6.3.3 Trello and Asana

Project management apps like Asana and Trello, which enable groups to assign roles, keep track of due dates, and assess progress, are examples of collaboration tools. Project management apps like Asana and Trello can be combined with design-thinking. Teams can assign responsibilities to members, set deadlines, and prioritize and organize tasks using these tools.

Trello is a visual board system that facilitates team collaboration and progress tracking by letting users make lists, cards, and boards. Card features like labels, attachments, and comments allow users to easily share ideas and feedback. A comparable feature set is provided by Asana, which includes task management, project tracking, and team collaboration. It also has a timeline function that lets users see dependencies and deadlines for projects.

Asana and Trello can both be integrated with other tools for collaboration, like Figma, so teams can move between project management and design work with ease. Through the combination of these tools with design-thinking, teams can guarantee that their projects are efficiently planned, effectively executed, and finished on schedule. All things considered, collaboration tools are critical to design-thinking because they facilitate more productive and successful cross-functional teamwork. Teams can generate ideas, prototype, and test solutions that satisfy user needs and produce significant results by utilizing these tools.

5.6.4 3D Printing Tools

Design-thinking can make use of 3D printing technologies to materialize concepts. With the aid of these tools, teams can quickly and simply produce physical prototypes of their designs, which can aid in the overall design's improvement. Below are a few instances of 3D printing tools:

- **Desktop 3D Printers:** teams of varying sizes and skill levels can utilize desktop 3D printers due to their accessibility and ease of use. Rather than relying on costly manufacturing equipment or outsourcing, teams can produce tangible prototypes of their designs internally using a desktop 3D printer.
- 3D **Scanner:** using 3D scanners, groups can scan real-world objects to produce digital models that can be enhanced and changed. Teams may need to make unique components that blend in perfectly with already-existing products, which is where this tool can be especially helpful in product design.
- **Ultimaker Cura:** Design thinkers can prepare their 3D models for printing with free and open-source software called Ultimaker Cura. To assist designers in making their designs more print-friendly, the software provides functions like model rotation, scaling, and support generation.
- **Autodesk Fusion 360:** design thinkers can create and edit 3D models, simulate designs, and generate toolpaths for 3D printing with Autodesk Fusion 360, a cloud-based 3D CAD/CAM tool. It provides tools like mesh editing and parametric modeling to assist designers in producing intricate, accurate designs.

In conclusion, teams can upload their designs to online 3D printing services, which then print and ship the finished products straight to them. Without the need for specialist tools or knowledge, these services' extensive selection of materials and finishes enables teams to quickly produce high-quality prototypes.

5.6.5 Data Visualization Tools

Data visualization tools can assist teams in making sense of complex data and information when applying Design-thinking principles. These tools enable teams to create visual representations of data, such as charts, graphs, and diagrams, which can aid in identifying patterns, trends, and insights. Some examples of data visualization tools include:

- Tableau: teams can connect to multiple data sources and generate interactive dashboards and reports with Tableau, a potent data visualization tool. Teams can swiftly explore and analyze large datasets with Tableau, spot trends, and patterns, and communicate their results to others.
- Infogram: graphs, infographics, and charts can be easily created by teams using Infogram, an online tool that eliminates the need for specialized design knowledge. Teams can easily visualize complex data and share their insights with others in a visually appealing way by using Infogram.
- Google Data Studio: design thinkers can create custom reports and dashboards using Google Analytics, Google Sheets, BigQuery, and other data sources with Google Data Studio, a free tool for data visualization. Design thinkers can use features like data filtering, customizing charts, and real-time collaboration to visualize and communicate insights with their teams.

All things considered, data visualization tools are a crucial component of the Design-thinking process because they enable teams to make sense of complicated data and effectively and persuasively convey their conclusions. Teams can produce more comprehensive results and make more comprehensive decisions for their users by utilizing these tools.

5.7 Conclusion

This chapter has discussed various tools and techniques that are used to develop user-centric design. Design-thinking requires a wide variety of tools to solve each phase of the Design-thinking cycle. In addition, we have looked at some popular techniques in the latter portions of this chapter.

References

Bruton, L. 2022. The benefits of a/b testing. https:// www.uxdesigninstitute.com/blog/benefits-of-a-b-testing/. (Accessed: January 23, 2024).

Cui, S. 2018. A guide to paper-prototype sketching. https://xinyicui.medium.com/ui-ux-strategy-a-guide-to-paper-prototype-sketching 3c475ce560f9#:~:text=Sketching%20can%20be%20used%20in,see%20if%20it%20has%20value. (Accessed: October 19, 2018).

Dam, R.F. and Teo, Y.S. 2016. 5 common low-fidelity prototypes and their best practices. https://www.interaction-design.org/literature/article/prototyping-learn-eight-common-methods-and-best-practices. (Accessed: January 10, 2024).

Dehant, B. 2023. Design thinking and workshops in VR (virtual reality). https://www.innovationtraining.org/virtual-reality-design-thinking-workshops-in-vr/. (Accessed: September 9, 2023).

Elmansy, R. 2023. How to apply 5 whys root cause analysis. https://www.designorate.com/how-to-apply-root-cause-analysis-using-5-whys/. (Accessed: January 17, 2024).

Gibbons, S . 2019. User need statements: The 'define' stage in design thinking. https://www.nngroup.com/articles/user-need-statements/. (Accessed: January 07, 2023).

Goulbourne, C.P. 2019. How empathy mapping can be used to help generate ideas for your business. https://obaninternational.com/ blog/empathy-mapping/. (Accessed: June 19, 2023).

Hotjar. 2023. Usability testing: what it is, benefits, and what it isn't. https://www.hotjar.com/usability-testing/. (Accessed: July 17, 2024).

Lewis, S. 2020. Fishbone diagram (ishikawa cause and effect). https://www.techtarget.com/whatis/definition/fishbone-diagram#:~:text=A%20fishbone%20diagram%20is%20a,type%20of%20mind%20map%20template. (Accessed: January 3, 2024).

Lewrick, M. and Link, P. and Leifer, L. 2018. The design Thinking Playbook: Mindful Digital Transformation of Teams, Products, Services, Businesses and Ecosystems. John Wiley & Sons.

Liedtka, J. and Ogilvie, T. 2011. Designing for Growth: A Design Thinking Tool Kit for Managers. Columbia University Press.

McCay, A. 2023a. Creating a persona—a step-by-step guide with tips and examples. https://uxpressia.com/blog/how-to-create-persona-guide examples. (Accessed: January 1, 2024).

McCay, A. 2023b. Customer journey mapping guide for beginners. https://uxpressia.com/blog/customer-journey-map-guide-examples. (Accessed: January 6, 2024).

Müller-Roterberg, C. 2020. Design thinking for dummies. John Wiley & Sons.

O'Donoghue, J. 2023. Ux personas pros and cons: pointless or powerful. https://makeiterate.com/ux-personas-pros-and-cons-pointless-or-powerful/#:~:text=Personas%20can%20give%20the%20illusion,ensure%20the%20personas%20remain%20accurate. (Accessed: January 1, 2024)

Pojasek, R.B. 2000. Asking "why?" five times. Environmental Quality Management. 10(1): 79–84.

Rojas, J. 2023. Learn how to use sketching as an ideation method. interaction design foundation - ixdf. https://www.interaction-design.org/literature/article/etch-a-sketch-how-to-use-sketching-in-user-experience-design. (Accessed: January 10, 2024).

Snyder, C. 2003. Paper Prototyping: The Fast and Easy Way to Design and Refine User Interfaces. Morgan Kaufmann.

Torsten, T. 2019. User testing: definition, how to, tools, methods. https://userpeek.com/blog/user-experience-testing/. (Accessed: January 11, 2024).

Chapter 6

Challenges and Pitfalls

The previous chapters have covered design-thinking in great detail, and it is clear that the method is effective for solving problems and can assist groups in developing novel solutions to challenging issues. Nevertheless, this methodology is not without its challenges and pitfalls. The following are some common challenges that teams face when implementing design-thinking techniques, (The Knowledge Academy, 2023):

- Lack of Empathy
- Poor Problem Definition
- Limited Ideation
- Inadequate Prototyping
- Insufficient Testing
- Bias and Assumptions
- Fears and Phobias
- Design Constraints
- Resistance to Change
- Lack of Cross-Functional Collaboration

6.1 Lack of Empathy

Design-thinking relies heavily on understanding the needs and perspectives of users or customers. However, it can be challenging to truly empathize with others, especially if they have different backgrounds or experiences. Without genuine empathy, the solutions generated may not effectively address user needs.

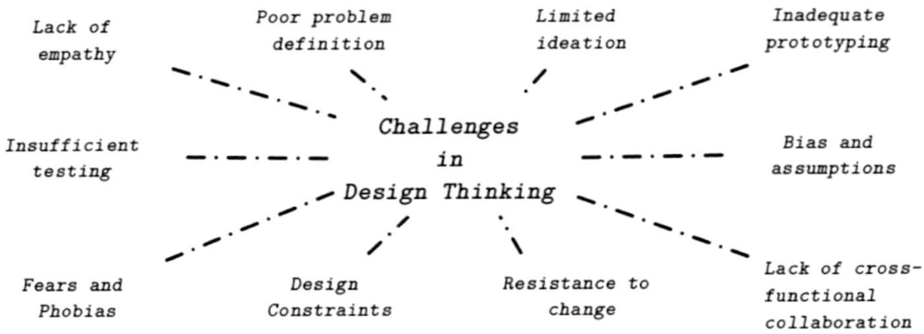

Figure 6.1: Challenges and Pitfalls in Design-Thinking

Lack of empathy in design-thinking refers to the failure to understand and consider the needs, wants, and perspectives of end-users or customers. It means that designers cannot empathize with the users and their experiences, which can result in solutions that do not meet their needs or solve their problems. This can lead to a lack of user engagement and satisfaction, resulting in poor product adoption and ultimately, failure in the market. Therefore, empathy is a critical component of design-thinking, as it helps designers understand the users' needs and create relevant solutions and effective (Clarke, Jodi, 2023). There are two types of empathy in design-thinking; cognitive empathy and emotional empathy:

6.1.1 Cognitive Empathy

Cognitive empathy is the ability to understand how others think and feel. Designers may lack cognitive empathy if they hold preconceived notions or biases that prevent them from understanding their users' needs and perspectives. A designer who creates a new mobile app for a bank without considering the user's needs and motivations exemplifies a lack of cognitive empathy in design-thinking. The designer may have focused solely on the technical aspects of the app, ignoring the user experience. As a result, the app is perhaps difficult to use, confusing, and frustrating for users. The designer may not have considered the user's thought process, such as their desire for simplicity and ease of use when managing their finances.

Lacking cognitive empathy, the designer may not understand that users are perhaps overwhelmed by complex financial jargon or require guidance to make informed financial decisions. As a result, the app may not be able to attract and retain users. A lack of cognitive empathy in design-thinking can result in products that fail to meet users' needs and expectations, leading to poor user experiences and low adoption rates.

6.1.2 Emotional Empathy

Emotional empathy refers to the ability to feel and respond to the emotions of others. Designers may lack emotional empathy if they are more focused on creating innovative or unique solutions than addressing the actual needs of users. An example of a lack of emotional empathy in design-thinking could be a designer who creates a new fitness app that encourages users to track their progress and set goals. However, the designer may overlook the emotional needs of users who may struggle with motivation or self-esteem issues related to their fitness journey.

The designer may have overlooked the fact that some users may feel discouraged or overwhelmed when they do not see immediate results or may feel demotivated when they compare themselves to others on the app. Without emotional empathy, the designer may not have considered how these emotions could impact the user's experience and motivation to continue using the app.

As a result, the app may not provide adequate support or encouragement for users who need emotional support and guidance. The designer may have focused solely on the technical aspects of the app, such as tracking progress and setting goals, without considering the emotional needs of users.

Overall, a lack of emotional empathy in design-thinking can lead to products that do not provide adequate emotional support for users, resulting in low engagement and retention rates.

6.1.3 Cognitive Empathy vs Emotional Empathy

Cognitive and emotional are two different types of empathy that can be applied in design-thinking.

Table 6.1: Cognitive Empathy vs Emotional Empathy

Cognitive Empathy	Emotional Empathy
Ability to understand and share someone else's perspective, thoughts, and feelings without necessarily feeling the same emotions.	Ability to feel and share the same emotions as someone else.
Can be used to understand the needs, goals, and motivations of users by observing their behavior, conducting user research, and analyzing data.	Can be used to understand the emotional needs of users and create products that provide emotional support and guidance.
Can help designers create products that meet the functional and practical needs of users.	Can help designers create products that are not only functional but also emotionally satisfying and meaningful for users.

Both types of empathy are important in design-thinking, as they help designers understand the needs and desires of users from different perspectives.

A balance of cognitive and emotional empathy can result in products that are not only functional but also emotionally engaging and satisfying.

6.2 Poor Problem Definition

The design-thinking process is perhaps hampered by overly general or restrictive problem definitions. A problem statement that is too specific may stifle creativity, while one that is too vague may result in solutions that fall short. Poor problem definition in design-thinking can lead to a variety of issues, including:

- **Lack of Clarity:** if the problem is not well-defined, stakeholders and team members may become uncertain about the issues that require attention.
- **Ineffective Solutions:** without a thorough understanding of the problem, the solutions developed might not adequately address the root cause or satisfy the users' needs.
- **Wasted Time and Resources:** poor problem definition can result in wasted time and resources as teams may work on solving the incorrect problem or go back and forth trying to clarify the issue.
- **Opportunities Lost:** due to the inability to identify the real problems or areas for expansion, a vague problem definition may lead to missed chances for innovation or improvement.
- **Lack of Stakeholder Buy-In:** when the problem is unclear, stakeholders may not fully understand or support the proposed solutions, leading to resistance and implementation challenges.

An example of poor problem definition in design-thinking could be a team tasked with improving customer satisfaction for a retail company. If the problem is defined too broadly as "increase customer satisfaction," the team may struggle to generate focused and actionable ideas during the ideation phase.

Without a clear understanding of customers' specific pain points and needs, the team may end up brainstorming generic solutions that fail to address the root causes of dissatisfaction. This can lead to wasted time and resources on ideas that do not effectively solve the problem.

To improve problem definition in this scenario, the team could conduct user research to identify key issues affecting customer satisfaction, such as long wait times at checkout, difficulty finding products, or poor customer service. By narrowing down the problem statement to something more specific, like "reduce wait times at checkout to improve customer satisfaction," the team can focus their ideation efforts on generating targeted solutions that directly address the identified pain point.

6.3 Limited Ideation

The consequence of limited ideation in design-thinking can significantly impact the overall quality and effectiveness of the design process. Limited ideation in design-thinking can lead to a variety of issues, including:

- **Narrow Solutions:** limited ideation can result in a narrow range of solutions being considered, leading to missed opportunities for innovative and creative ideas. This can limit the potential for breakthrough solutions that address the root causes of a problem.
- **Lack of Differentiation:** when ideation is constrained, it can lead to solutions that are similar to existing products or services in the market. This lack of differentiation can hinder a design's ability to stand out and meet the unique needs of users.
- **Missed Opportunities:** limited ideation may prevent teams from exploring alternative perspectives or considering unconventional ideas that could lead to novel solutions. This can result in missed opportunities to address user needs in innovative ways.
- **Reduced Engagement:** when team members feel their ideas are not valued or that they are unable to contribute during ideation sessions, it can lead to disengagement and reduced motivation. This can impact the overall collaboration and creativity of the team.
- **Ineffective Problem-Solving:** design-thinking relies on a robust ideation process to generate a diverse set of ideas that can be evaluated and refined to solve complex problems. Limited ideation can impede the problem-solving process and result in suboptimal solutions.
- **Decreased Innovation:** design-thinking is rooted in innovation and creativity, and limited ideation can stifle the generation of truly innovative ideas. Without a wide range of ideas to draw from, teams may struggle to push the boundaries of what is possible and create truly transformative solutions.

Limited ideation in design-thinking can occur when a team only generates a few ideas or fails to explore a wide range of possibilities. For instance, a team working on designing a new mobile app for fitness tracking may conduct an ideation session but only come up with a handful of ideas, such as tracking steps, calories burned, and distance covered.

This limited ideation approach can hinder the team's ability to consider innovative and creative solutions that could set their app apart from competitors. By restricting their brainstorming to a few obvious features, the team may miss out on opportunities to address unmet user needs or introduce unique functionalities that could make the app more appealing and user-friendly.

By expanding their ideation process and exploring a wide range of possibilities, teams can uncover innovative solutions that address user needs more effectively and differentiate their designs in the market.

6.4 Inadequate Prototyping

Inadequate prototyping in design-thinking can occur when a team rushes through the prototyping phase or fails to create prototypes that effectively test and iterate on their ideas. For example, a team working on designing a new website for an e-commerce platform may quickly create a basic wireframe prototype without considering user interaction, functionality, or visual design elements. This lack of attention to detail in prototyping can lead to several issues that hinder the design process and the ultimate success of the product. Some consequences of inadequate prototyping include:

- **Failure to Uncover Usability Issues:** without thorough prototyping, teams may miss critical usability issues that could impact the user experience. Inadequate prototypes may not accurately simulate user interactions, leading to overlooked problems that could have been addressed early on.
- **Limited Feedback and Validation:** inadequate prototypes may not provide stakeholders and users with a clear representation of the final product, making it difficult to gather meaningful feedback and validate design decisions. This can result in missed opportunities for improvement and refinement.
- **Ineffective Communication:** prototypes serve as a communication tool to convey design concepts and ideas to stakeholders and team members. Inadequate prototypes may fail to effectively communicate the vision and functionality of the design, leading to misunderstandings and misalignment among team members.

By improving the quality and effectiveness of prototypes in the design-thinking process, teams can enhance their ability to innovate, validate ideas, and create successful products that meet user needs.

6.5 Insufficient Testing

Insufficient testing in design-thinking can occur when a team fails to conduct thorough and meaningful testing to validate their ideas, gather feedback, and iterate on their designs. This lack of testing can lead to several challenges and drawbacks that hinder the success of the design process and the final product. Some consequences of insufficient testing include:

- **Unidentified Usability Issues:** without comprehensive testing, teams may overlook critical usability issues that could impact the user experience. Failure to test prototypes with real users can result in missed opportunities to identify and address usability problems early on.
- **Limited Validation of Design Decisions:** insufficient testing may prevent teams from validating their design decisions and assumptions with real users. Without feedback from users, stakeholders, or experts, teams may struggle to assess the effectiveness of their designs and make informed decisions for improvement.
- **Inaccurate Assumptions:** without testing, teams may rely on assumptions about user behavior, preferences, and needs, leading to design solutions that do not align with actual user expectations. Testing helps validate these assumptions and ensures that designs are based on real user insights.
- **Missed Opportunities for Iteration:** testing is essential for gathering feedback, identifying areas for improvement, and iterating on design solutions. Insufficient testing may result in missed opportunities to refine and enhance designs based on user feedback, leading to suboptimal outcomes.

By prioritizing thorough testing in the design-thinking process, teams can ensure that their designs are user-centered, validated, and optimized for success. Testing is a critical step in the design process that helps teams create products that meet user needs and deliver value.

6.6 Bias and Assumptions

Designers may unknowingly bring their own biases and assumptions into the design process, which can limit their ability to see alternative perspectives or solutions. It is important to challenge these biases and actively seek diverse viewpoints to ensure a more inclusive and comprehensive approach. There are several types of bias and assumptions in design-thinking, (NSHCS., 2019):

6.6.1 Confirmation Bias

Confirmation bias refers to the tendency to seek out information that confirms preexisting beliefs or assumptions while ignoring information that contradicts them. Confirmation bias in design-thinking refers to the tendency of designers to seek out information that confirms their existing beliefs or assumptions while ignoring or downplaying information that contradicts their beliefs. This can lead to a narrow focus on a particular solution or approach and prevent designers from considering alternative ideas or perspectives.

Confirmation bias can occur at any stage of the design-thinking process, from problem definition to ideation, prototyping, and testing. For example, a designer may define a problem too narrowly based on their own experiences or assumptions, or they may only test their prototype with users who are likely to confirm their design choices.

To avoid confirmation bias in design-thinking, designers could benefit greatly from actively seeking out diverse perspectives and feedback throughout the process. This can involve conducting user research with a wide range of users, engaging in collaborative brainstorming sessions with team members from different backgrounds and disciplines, and testing prototypes with a diverse group of users to identify any potential biases or limitations in the design.

6.6.2 Affinity Bias

Affinity bias in design-thinking refers to the tendency of designers to favor or be more comfortable with people who share similar backgrounds, experiences, or perspectives as themselves. This can lead to a lack of diversity in the design team and a narrow focus on solutions that may only work for a specific group of users.

Affinity bias can occur at any stage of the design-thinking process, from problem definition to ideation, prototyping, and testing. For example, a design team may only recruit members who have similar educational backgrounds or work experiences or may only test their prototypes with users who are similar to themselves.

To avoid affinity bias in design-thinking, designers could benefit greatly from actively seeking out diverse perspectives and feedback throughout the process. This can involve recruiting team members from different backgrounds and disciplines, conducting user research with a wide range of users, and testing prototypes with a diverse group of users to identify any potential biases or limitations in the design. Additionally, designers should be aware of their own biases and actively work to challenge them by seeking out new perspectives and experiences.

6.6.3 Attribution Bias

Attribution bias in design-thinking refers to the tendency of designers to attribute the successes or failures of a design project to internal or external factors rather than considering the full range of factors that may have contributed to the outcome.

For example, a design team may attribute the success of a project solely to their skills and expertise, ignoring external factors such as luck or market conditions that may have played a role. Similarly, a team may blame external factors such as budget constraints or time limitations for a project's failure without considering whether their own design decisions or processes may have contributed to the outcome.

To avoid attribution bias in design-thinking, designers could benefit greatly from accepting a holistic approach to evaluating the success or failure of a project. This can involve considering a range of factors that may have contributed to the outcome, including internal and external factors, as well as the design process itself. Designers could benefit greatly from also being willing to take responsibility for their own decisions and actions and be open to feedback and criticism to improve their future work.

6.6.4 Beauty Bias

Beauty bias in design-thinking refers to the tendency of designers to prioritize aesthetics over functionality or usability in their designs. This bias can lead to designs that may look visually appealing but may not necessarily meet the needs or preferences of the intended users.

For example, a designer may focus on creating a visually stunning website or app but may overlook important usability features such as clear navigation or easy-to-use interfaces. This can result in a design that is aesthetically pleasing but frustrating for users to navigate.

To avoid beauty bias in design-thinking, designers could benefit greatly from prioritizing function and usability over aesthetics. This can involve conducting user research to understand the needs and preferences of the target audience and incorporating these insights into the design process. Designers should also be willing to iterate and test their designs with users to ensure that they are not only visually appealing but also functional and usable.

6.6.5 Conformity Bias

Conformity bias in design-thinking refers to the tendency of designers to conform to existing design standards or trends rather than exploring new and innovative ideas. This bias can limit creativity and innovation in the design process, as designers are perhaps hesitant to deviate from established norms or risk trying something new.

For example, a designer may conform to the standard layout and design of a website or app, rather than exploring new and potentially more effective ways of organizing information or presenting content. This can result in a design that is perhaps functional but lacks creativity and innovation.

To avoid conformity bias in design-thinking, designers could benefit greatly from challenging existing design standards and exploring new ideas and approaches. This can involve conducting research on emerging design trends and technologies, as well as seeking feedback from users and stakeholders to understand their needs and preferences. Designers should also be willing to take risks and try new things, even if they do not conform to established norms or standards.

6.6.6 Gender Bias

Gender bias in design-thinking refers to the tendency of designers to create products, services, or experiences that are biased towards one gender, often based on stereotypes and assumptions. This can lead to exclusion, discrimination, and a lack of diversity in design.

For example, a product designed for women is perhaps assumed to be pink and feminine, while a product designed for men is perhaps assumed to be rugged and masculine. This can limit the choices available to consumers and perpetuate gender stereotypes.

To avoid gender bias in design-thinking, designers could benefit greatly from striving for inclusivity and diversity in their design process. This can involve conducting research and gathering feedback from a diverse group of users, considering the needs and preferences of different genders, and avoiding assumptions and stereotypes. Designers should also be aware of the impact of their designs on different genders and work towards creating products and services that are accessible and inclusive for all.

6.6.7 The Halo Effect

The *halo effect* in design-thinking refers to the cognitive bias where a positive impression of a product, service, or brand influences a person's overall perception and evaluation of that entity. This bias can lead to overestimating the strengths and capabilities of the entity while overlooking or minimizing its weaknesses and limitations.

In design-thinking, the halo effect can impact the design process by causing designers to focus too much on the positive aspects of their designs while neglecting potential flaws or areas for improvement. This can result in a lack of critical evaluation and feedback, which can ultimately lead to a less effective or successful product or service.

To avoid the halo effect in design-thinking, designers could benefit greatly from striving for objectivity and critical evaluation throughout the design process. This can involve seeking out diverse perspectives and feedback, conducting thorough research and testing, and being open to constructive criticism and suggestions for improvement. By remaining mindful of the potential for bias and actively working to counteract it, designers can create more effective and impactful designs.

6.6.8 Contrast Effect

The contrast effect in design-thinking refers to the cognitive bias where a person's perception of a product, service, or brand is influenced by the comparison to a similar entity that was experienced immediately beforehand. This bias can cause the person to either overestimate or underestimate the qualities of the entity based on the comparison.

In design-thinking, the contrast effect can impact the design process by causing designers to focus too much on the differences between their design and a competitor's design, rather than evaluating their design on its own merits. This can lead to a design that is overly influenced by the competition, rather than being a unique and effective solution for the user's needs.

To avoid the contrast effect in design-thinking, designers could benefit greatly from striving to evaluate their designs objectively and independently of any comparisons to competitors. This can involve conducting user research and testing to understand the user's needs and preferences and using this information to inform the design process. By focusing on the user's needs and goals, rather than the competition, designers can create more effective and impactful designs.

6.6.9 Ageism

Ageism in design-thinking refers to the discrimination or bias against individuals based on their age, particularly in the design of products, services, or experiences. This bias can manifest in various ways, such as assuming that older individuals are less tech-savvy or less interested in new products, or designing products that cater only to younger demographics.

Ageism in design-thinking can have negative consequences, such as excluding older individuals from important products and services or creating products that are difficult for them to use. This can lead to frustration, isolation, and a lack of access to essential resources.

To combat ageism in design-thinking, designers could benefit greatly from striving to understand the needs and preferences of all age groups, including older individuals. This can involve conducting user research and testing with diverse age groups, designing products that are inclusive and accessible to all users, and avoiding assumptions based on age stereotypes. By embracing diversity and inclusivity in design-thinking, designers can create products and services that meet the needs of all users, regardless of age.

6.6.10 Name bias

Name bias in design-thinking refers to the discrimination or bias against individuals based on their name, particularly in the design of products, services, or experiences. This bias can manifest in various ways, such as assuming certain names are associated with certain ethnicities or cultures, or designing products that cater only to certain names or name spellings.

Name bias in design-thinking can have negative consequences, such as excluding individuals with certain names from important products and services or creating products that are difficult for them to use. This can lead to frustration, isolation, and a lack of access to essential resources.

To combat name bias in design-thinking, designers could benefit greatly from striving to understand the needs and preferences of all individuals, regardless of their names. This can involve conducting user research and testing with diverse groups of people, designing products that are inclusive and accessible to all users, and avoiding assumptions based on name stereotypes. By embracing diversity and inclusivity in design-thinking, designers can create products and services that meet the needs of all users, regardless of their name.

6.7 Fears and Phobias

Fear is a common emotion that can arise during the design-thinking process(Beaver, C, 2023). Some common fears that designers may experience include:

6.7.1 Fear of Failure

The fear of failure in design-thinking can be a significant obstacle for designers. This fear can prevent designers from taking risks and trying new ideas, which can limit their creativity and the potential success of their solutions. Designers may fear failure because they worry about negative feedback or consequences, such as losing their jobs or damaging their reputation. However, failure is a natural part of the design-thinking process, and it is essential to embrace this reality to achieve success.

To overcome the fear of failure in design-thinking, designers could benefit greatly from adopting a growth mindset. This involves recognizing that failure is an opportunity for learning and growth. By reframing failure as a necessary step toward success, designers can approach their work with more confidence and creativity. It would also be very beneficial to concentrate on the process rather than the product, realizing that every trial and error is an important step on the path to a good solution.

Designers can also overcome the fear of failure by seeking feedback from others. By sharing their work with colleagues and stakeholders, valuable insights and perspectives can be gained that can help them improve their solutions. Finally, designers could benefit greatly from remembering that failure is not a reflection of their worth or abilities as designers. Instead, it is an opportunity to learn, grow, and create more comprehensive solutions in the future.

6.7.2 Fear of Criticism

This refers to the fear of receiving negative feedback or criticism of one's designs or ideas. Fear of criticism is a common concern in design-thinking, especially during the ideation and prototyping phases. Designers often fear that their ideas or designs will be criticized or rejected by others, which can lead to a lack of confidence and hesitation in pursuing their ideas.

It is crucial to keep in mind, though, that feedback is a normal component of the design process and can help to enhance the finished item. Instead of viewing criticism and comments as a personal jab at their knowledge or abilities, designers would tremendously benefit from viewing them as opportunities to grow and learn.

6.7.3 Fear of Rejection

The fear of rejection in design-thinking is the fear of being criticized, dismissed, or rejected by stakeholders for the ideas and solutions that a designer presents. Designers may experience this fear because they want to create solutions that are accepted and embraced by stakeholders, and they may feel pressure to come up with ideas that meet everyone's expectations. This fear can lead to designers holding back their ideas or not taking risks, which can hinder the creative process and lead to less effective solutions. Overcoming the fear of rejection in design-thinking involves building confidence, embracing feedback, and reframing rejection as a natural part of the process.

6.7.4 Fear of Making Mistakes or 'Atelophobia'

This refers to the fear of making errors or mistakes in the design process, which can lead to wasted time and resources. The fear of making mistakes in design-thinking is the fear of failure or producing something that is not up to standard. Designers may experience this fear because they want to create perfect solutions and avoid any negative feedback or consequences. This fear can lead to designers being overly cautious, which can hinder the creative process and prevent them from exploring new ideas and taking risks. Overcoming the fear of making mistakes in design-thinking involves embracing a growth mindset, accepting that mistakes are a natural part of the process, and learning from them to improve future solutions. Designers could also benefit from focusing on the process rather than just the outcome and being willing to experiment and iterate until they find the strongest possible solution.

6.7.5 Fear of the Unknown

The fear of the unknown can be a significant obstacle to design-thinking. This fear can prevent designers from exploring new ideas and taking risks, which can limit their creativity and the potential success of their solutions. Designers may fear the unknown because they worry about the uncertainty of the outcome or the potential risks involved.

To overcome the fear of the unknown in design-thinking, designers could benefit greatly from embracing curiosity and exploration. This involves being open to new ideas and perspectives and actively seeking out opportunities to learn and discover. Designers should also be willing to take calculated risks, recognizing that failure is a natural part of the design-thinking process.

Designers can also overcome the fear of the unknown by breaking down complex problems into smaller, more manageable parts. This can help them identify areas of uncertainty and develop strategies for addressing them. Additionally, designers can collaborate with others to gain different perspectives and insights, which can help reduce the fear of the unknown.

Finally, designers could benefit greatly from remembering that the unknown is not always negative. It can often lead to discoveries and innovative solutions. By embracing the unknown and seeing it as an opportunity rather than a threat, designers can unlock their creativity and achieve greater success in their work.

6.7.6 Loss of Control

Fear of losing control over one's work or personal life can be a significant factor contributing to resistance to change. When individuals feel like they are losing control over their work processes, projects, or personal decisions, they may resist changes that disrupt their sense of autonomy and stability.

Change often involves shifts in roles, responsibilities, or decision-making processes that can diminish individuals' sense of autonomy and independence. When people fear losing control over their work or personal lives, they may resist changes that limit their ability to make choices or have a say in important decisions.

Change introduces uncertainty and unpredictability into people's lives, which can be unsettling for those who value stability and predictability. The fear of not knowing what the future holds or how changes will impact one's work or personal life can lead to resistance to change.

Change can bring new challenges, risks, and growth opportunities, but it also carries the risk of failure. Individuals who fear making mistakes, facing criticism, or not meeting expectations may resist changes that require them to step outside their comfort zone and take on new responsibilities.

Change often triggers emotional responses such as anxiety, stress, or fear of the unknown. People may resist change because they are not comfortable with the emotions that come with navigating uncertainty, adapting to new circumstances, or letting go of familiar routines.

To address resistance to change related to the fear of losing control, organizations and individuals can take proactive steps to build resilience, foster adaptability, and cultivate a growth mindset. Providing support, resources, and opportunities for learning and development can help individuals feel more confident and capable of navigating change. Encouraging open communication, transparency, and collaboration can also help alleviate fears and concerns related to losing control over work or personal life. By acknowledging and addressing the underlying fears and anxieties that drive resistance to change, individuals can embrace new opportunities for growth, innovation, and personal development.

6.8 Design Constraints

Design constraints are limitations or restrictions imposed by both internal and external factors during the design process. Everybody in the company needs to be aware of these limitations and take them into account before beginning any project because they affect the finished product. Several common types of design constraints were proposed by UXPin (2023), which include:

6.8.1 Technical Constraints

Technical constraints in design-thinking refer to limitations or restrictions imposed by the available technology, resources, or technical specifications that may impact the design process and outcomes. These constraints can influence the feasibility, functionality, usability, and overall success of a design solution. Some examples of technical constraints in design-thinking are:

- **Screen Size and Resolution:** different devices have varying screen sizes and resolutions, which can affect the layout and visual presentation of the user interface. Designers need to create responsive designs that adapt to different screen sizes to ensure a consistent and user-friendly experience across devices.
- **Input Methods:** devices may have different input methods, such as touchscreens, keyboards, or voice commands. Designers must consider these input methods when designing interactions and navigation within the app to accommodate various user preferences and device capabilities.
- **Performance:** older devices or those with limited hardware capabilities may struggle to run complex or resource-intensive applications smoothly. Designers need to optimize their designs for performance by minimizing unnecessary animations, graphics, or features that could slow down the app on certain devices.

- **Operating System Compatibility:** different operating systems (e.g., iOS, Android) have unique design guidelines, interactions, and restrictions. Designers must adhere to these guidelines to ensure consistency and usability across platforms while also considering platform-specific features and limitations.
- **Accessibility:** device and operating system limitations can impact the accessibility of digital products for users with disabilities. Designers need to consider accessibility standards and guidelines to ensure that their designs are inclusive and usable for all users, regardless of their device or operating system.

By understanding and addressing device and operating system limitations in the design process, designers can create more effective and user-centric digital products that provide a seamless experience across various devices and platforms. Collaboration with developers and testing on different devices can help identify and overcome these constraints to deliver a successful design solution.

6.8.2 Financial Constraints

Financial constraints play a significant role in design-thinking, as they can impact the resources available for research, prototyping, testing, and implementation of design solutions. Designers often need to work within budget limitations to deliver innovative and effective solutions that meet the needs of users and stakeholders. Here are some ways in which financial constraints can influence design-thinking:

- A limited budget may require designers to prioritize resources and focus on high-impact design decisions that align with project goals and constraints. Designers must make strategic choices about where to allocate funds to maximize the value of the design solution.
- Developing prototypes is a crucial part of the design process to test and iterate on ideas before final implementation. Financial constraints may limit the scope or fidelity of prototypes, requiring designers to find cost-effective ways to validate concepts and gather feedback from users.
- Conducting user research is essential for understanding user needs, behaviors, and preferences. Financial constraints may restrict the budget for user research activities, such as interviews, surveys, or usability testing. Designers must find creative and affordable methods to gather insights and validate assumptions.
- Design solutions often involve physical materials, technology components, or software licenses that incur costs. Designers need to consider the cost of materials and technologies when developing prototypes or

implementing final products, balancing quality and functionality with budget constraints.

- Design solutions should be scalable and sustainable over time, considering future updates, maintenance, and support costs. Designers must factor in ongoing expenses related to maintenance, updates, and user support when designing products within financial constraints.

Despite financial limitations, designers can leverage design-thinking principles to innovate and create impactful solutions within budget constraints. By focusing on user needs, collaboration with stakeholders, iterative prototyping, and efficient resource management, designers can overcome financial challenges and deliver successful design outcomes that drive value for users and businesses alike.

6.8.3 Legal and Regulatory Constraints

Legal and regulatory constraints play a crucial role in design-thinking, as they define the boundaries within which designers must operate to ensure compliance with laws, regulations, and industry standards. Designers need to consider legal and regulatory requirements throughout the design process to mitigate risks, protect users, and uphold ethical standards. Here are some ways in which legal and regulatory constraints can influence design-thinking:

- Designers must adhere to data privacy regulations, such as the General Data Protection Regulation (GDPR) in Europe or the California Consumer Privacy Act (CCPA) in the United States. They need to consider how user data is collected, stored, processed, and protected within their design solutions to ensure compliance with privacy laws.
- Designers must comply with accessibility standards, such as the Web Content Accessibility Guidelines (WCAG), to ensure that their products are usable by people with disabilities. They need to consider factors like screen reader compatibility, keyboard navigation, color contrast, and other accessibility features when designing digital interfaces.
- Designers need to respect intellectual property rights, including trademarks, copyrights, and patents when creating new products or services. They must avoid infringing on existing intellectual property and ensure that their designs do not violate the rights of others.
- Designers working on physical products or environments must consider health and safety regulations to protect users from potential hazards or risks. They need to conduct risk assessments, follow safety standards, and incorporate safety features into their designs to ensure user well-being.
- Designers could greatly benefit from considering the ethical implications of their design decisions, such as avoiding bias in algorithms, promoting

inclusivity and diversity, and respecting cultural sensitivities. They need to design ethically responsible solutions that prioritize user well-being and societal impact.

- Designers must be aware of industry-specific regulations and compliance requirements that may impact their design solutions. They need to work closely with legal experts and regulatory professionals to ensure that their designs meet all relevant standards and guidelines.

By considering legal and regulatory constraints early in the design process, designers can proactively address compliance issues, mitigate risks, and build trust with users and stakeholders. Collaboration with legal counsel, regulatory experts, and compliance officers is essential to navigate complex legal landscapes and ensure that design solutions meet all requirements. By integrating legal and regulatory considerations into design-thinking practices, designers can create innovative solutions that are not only user-centered but also legally compliant and ethically responsible.

6.8.4 Organizational Constraints

Organizational constraints can significantly impact the design-thinking process and shape the way designers approach problem-solving and innovation within a specific company or context. These constraints may include factors such as:

- Designers may face tight deadlines and time pressures that impact the design process. Rapid development cycles, product launch schedules, or market demands can limit the amount of time available for research, ideation, prototyping, and testing.
- The culture of an organization can either support or hinder design-thinking initiatives. A culture that values creativity, collaboration, risk-taking, and user-centered approaches can foster innovation, while a more hierarchical, risk-averse, or siloed culture may pose challenges to the design process.
- Designers need to navigate stakeholder expectations and align their design solutions with the goals and priorities of various stakeholders, including executives, product managers, marketing teams, and end-users. Balancing competing interests and managing stakeholder feedback can be a significant organizational constraint.
- Designers may have to work within existing systems, processes, or technologies that constrain their ability to innovate or implement new design solutions. Legacy systems can present technical challenges and limitations that impact the feasibility and scalability of design ideas.
- Organizational constraints related to legal and regulatory requirements, industry standards, and compliance obligations can influence the design

process. Designers must ensure that their solutions meet all relevant regulations and standards, which may require additional time, resources, and expertise.

- Effective collaboration and communication within cross-functional teams are essential for successful design-thinking. Organizational constraints related to team dynamics, conflicts, or lack of interdisciplinary collaboration can hinder the design process and limit the effectiveness of design solutions.

By acknowledging and addressing organizational constraints, designers can navigate challenges effectively, leverage opportunities for innovation, and drive positive change within their organizations through design-thinking practices.

6.8.5 Self-Imposed Constraints

Self-imposed constraints in design-thinking refer to intentional limitations or restrictions that designers choose to impose on themselves during the creative process. These constraints can serve as catalysts for innovation, creativity, and problem-solving by encouraging designers to think outside the box, focus on key priorities, and push the boundaries of their creativity. Some common self-imposed constraints in design-thinking include:

- Limiting the resources available for a design project, such as budget, materials, or tools, can spark creative problem-solving and encourage designers to find unconventional solutions. Working with limited resources forces designers to be resourceful, innovative, and efficient in their approach.
- Defining a narrow scope or specific problem statement for a design project can help focus the design process and prevent scope creep. By limiting the scope of the project, designers can concentrate on addressing key challenges and generating targeted solutions that meet user needs effectively.
- Intentionally restricting the use of certain technologies or tools can push designers to explore alternative methods, experiment with new techniques, and think creatively about how to achieve their design goals. Technology constraints can inspire innovative thinking and novel approaches to problem-solving.
- Working with limited materials or constraints related to material properties, availability, or sustainability can stimulate creativity and encourage designers to consider new materials, textures, or fabrication techniques. Material constraints can lead to unique design solutions that are environmentally friendly and resource-efficient.

- Imposing constraints related to cultural norms, values, or user preferences can challenge designers to consider diverse perspectives, cultural sensitivities, and inclusivity in their design solutions. Cultural constraints can inspire designers to create products that resonate with a specific audience or address cultural needs effectively.
- Collaborating with experts from different disciplines or industries can introduce constraints related to interdisciplinary communication, collaboration, and integration of diverse perspectives. Interdisciplinary constraints can foster cross-pollination of ideas, encourage knowledge sharing, and promote holistic problem-solving approaches.

By embracing self-imposed constraints in design-thinking, designers can enhance their creativity, innovation, and problem-solving skills. These constraints encourage designers to think critically, challenge assumptions, and explore unconventional solutions that push the boundaries of traditional design practices. Ultimately, self-imposed constraints can lead to breakthrough ideas, meaningful innovations, and impactful design solutions that address complex challenges effectively.

6.8.6 Talent Constraints

Talent constraints in design-thinking refer to limitations or challenges related to the skills, expertise, or capabilities of the design team members involved in a project. These constraints can impact the effectiveness of the design process and the quality of the design outcomes. Some common talent constraints in design-thinking include:

- Design teams may face talent constraints due to skill gaps or deficiencies in specific areas such as user research, prototyping, visual design, or storytelling. Lack of expertise in critical design disciplines can hinder the team's ability to generate innovative ideas, create user-centric solutions, or communicate effectively with stakeholders.
- Variations in experience levels among team members can create talent constraints in design-thinking. Junior designers may lack the experience and knowledge needed to tackle complex design challenges, while senior designers may struggle to adapt to new technologies or emerging trends. Balancing diverse experience levels within a team is crucial to overcoming talent constraints and fostering collaboration.
- Design projects often require specialized expertise in niche areas such as interaction design, service design, data visualization, or accessibility. Talent constraints may arise when the team lacks individuals with the specialized skills to effectively address specific project requirements. Collaborating with external experts or upskilling team members can help overcome these constraints.

- Limited creative diversity within the design team can lead to talent constraints in design-thinking. Homogeneous teams may struggle to generate diverse perspectives, innovative ideas, or out-of-the-box solutions. Encouraging diversity in terms of backgrounds, experiences, and perspectives can enrich the design process and mitigate talent constraints.
- Effective collaboration is essential for successful design-thinking, but talent constraints related to poor communication, teamwork, or conflict resolution skills can hinder collaboration within the design team. Building strong team dynamics, fostering open communication, and promoting a culture of collaboration can help overcome talent constraints and enhance the design process.
- Design teams must be adaptable and flexible in response to changing project requirements, stakeholder feedback, or market dynamics. Talent constraints related to a lack of adaptability or resistance to change can impede the team's ability to pivot quickly, iterate on ideas, and respond to evolving user needs. Cultivating a growth mindset and embracing experimentation can help mitigate these constraints.
- Effective leadership is critical for guiding the design process, aligning team members' goals, and driving innovation. Talent constraints related to a lack of leadership skills or vision can hinder the team's ability to stay focused, motivated, and aligned toward achieving project objectives. Developing leadership capabilities within the team can address these constraints.

By recognizing and addressing talent constraints in design-thinking, teams can enhance their problem-solving capabilities, foster creativity, and deliver impactful design solutions that meet user needs effectively. Investing in talent development, promoting continuous learning, and fostering a culture of collaboration can help mitigate talent constraints and empower design teams to achieve their full potential.

6.9 Resistance to Change

Resistance to change in design-thinking can be a common challenge that organizations and teams may face when implementing new design methodologies or approaches. As has been discussed, the fear of the unknown is the main reason for resistance to change(Spring, Kealy , 2021).

People may resist change because they are comfortable with the current design and do not want to disrupt their routine or work processes. Design-thinking often requires a shift in mindset and a willingness to embrace ambiguity and experimentation, which can be uncomfortable for those accustomed to more traditional ways of working.

Another reason for resistance to change is a lack of trust in the leadership team or the company as a whole. A lack of trust can have implications for turnover as well as employees giving leadership the benefit of the doubt when issues do arise. Employees who resist a change initiative are often responding more to the person in the leadership position than the change itself. This comes about if those in leadership positions have not yet earned the trust of the employees, like when there is a new leader within the organization. It can also come about as a result of previous experiences that have caused employees to distrust leadership.

6.9.1 Personal Factors

Personal factors such as personality traits, values, and prior experiences can all have a significant impact on an individual's resistance to change, even when it comes to design-thinking. Individuals with certain personality traits, such as a strong preference for consistency and regularity (e.g., high levels of conscientiousness), may be less open to changes in design-thinking. People who are particularly open to new experiences, on the other hand, may be more willing to accept novel concepts and methods. Personal values, such as a strong commitment to tradition or a focus on efficiency, can affect how people perceive and respond to changes in the design-thinking paradigm. Individuals who prioritize tradition over modern design methods, for example, might be less receptive to using them. Before experiencing both positive and negative change, an individual's attitudes toward change in design-thinking can be influenced. If a person has had a negative experience in the past with change initiatives, they may be less likely to adopt new strategies.

In addition to these, other elements like cognitive biases, which affect how people understand and react to novel ideas, can also cause resistance to change in design-thinking. Examples of these biases include confirmation bias, which favors information that supports preexisting beliefs, and anchoring bias, which places an undue emphasis on initial information.

Moreover, resistance to change in design-thinking may also be influenced by emotions like fear, anxiety, or discomfort. People are perhaps resistant to change because they perceive the uncertainty and possible risks that come with attempting new things as threats. Organizations can more comprehensively assist people in overcoming their reluctance and embracing new ways of thinking and working by comprehending and addressing these personal factors that contribute to resistance to change in design-thinking. Offering chances for learning, development, and assistance can assist people in acquiring the abilities and perspective required to successfully manage and adjust to change.

6.9.2 Inadequate Communication

Lack of proper communication is a common factor that can contribute to resistance to change. When individuals feel left in the dark, uninformed, or excluded from the decision-making process surrounding changes in their work environment or personal lives, they are perhaps more likely to resist those changes.

When information about upcoming changes is not communicated, consistently, or on time, it can create uncertainty and confusion among individuals. Without a clear understanding of why changes are happening, what they entail, and how they will impact them, people may feel anxious, unsettled, or resistant to the unknown.

Poor communication can erode trust and credibility between leaders, managers, and employees. When individuals feel that information is being withheld, misrepresented, or not shared openly and honestly, it can lead to skepticism, cynicism, and resistance to change initiatives. In addition, miscommunication or lack of communication can lead to a misalignment of expectations between different stakeholders involved in the change process. When individuals have different understandings or interpretations of the changes being implemented, it can create conflicts, misunderstandings, and resistance to moving forward.

Effective communication is essential for gaining buy-in and engagement from individuals affected by change. When leaders or decision-makers fail to communicate the rationale, benefits, and goals of proposed changes, people are perhaps less likely to support or actively participate in the change process.

6.10 Lack of Cross-Functional Collaboration

Lack of cross-functional collaboration in design-thinking can lead to siloed thinking, limited perspectives, and missed opportunities for innovation. When team members from different disciplines and backgrounds do not work together, they may not fully understand the problem or the user's needs, resulting in solutions that are not as effective or impactful. Cross-functional collaboration is essential in design-thinking to bring diverse perspectives, expertise, and skills to the table, leading to more creative and holistic solutions. Without it, organizations may struggle to create truly innovative and user-centered products and services.

6.11 Conclusion

Even though design-thinking offers a lot of advantages, to apply the methodology effectively, one must be aware of these potential obstacles and pitfalls. By being aware of these obstacles and traps, organizations and designers can make the most of the design-thinking process and enhance their capacity for creativity and problem-solving.

References

Clarke, Jodi. 2023. Cognitive empathy vs. emotional empathy. https://www.verywellmind.com/cognitive-and-emotional-empathy-4582389. (Accessed: January 30, 2023).

Beaver, C. 2023. How to improve your problem solving skills as a vp of strategy. https://advisorycloud.com/blog/how-to-improve-your-problem-solving-skills-as-a-vp-of-strategy. (Accessed: Accessed: February 24, 2024).

NSHCS. 2019. Understanding different types of bias—conscious inclusion—equality, diversity and inclusion—about. https://nshcs.hee.nhs.uk/ about/equality-diversity-and-inclusion/conscious-inclusion/understanding-different-types-of-bias/. (Accessed: July 17, 2024).

Spring, Kealy . 2021. Overcoming resistance to change within your organization. https://www.betterup.com/blog/resistance-to-change#:~:text=it%20more%20effectively.-,What%20is%20resistance%20to%20change%3F,in%20fear%20of%20the%20unknown. (Accessed: February 06, 2024).

The Knowledge Academy. 2023. Design thinking problems - how to find the problem with solutions? https://www.theknowledgeacademy.com/blog/design-thinking-problem/. (Accessed: February 14, 2024).

UXPin. 2023. 7 constraints in design and how to overcome them. https:// www.uxpin.com/studio/blog/constraints-in-design/. (Accessed: February 6, 2024).

Chapter 7

Design-Thinking to Futures-Thinking

Futures-thinking, or foresight is a strategic and systematic approach to anticipating and preparing for future trends, challenges, opportunities, and possibilities. It involves exploring different scenarios, analyzing potential outcomes, and envisioning alternative futures to inform decision-making and planning in the present. Futures-thinking goes beyond traditional forecasting by emphasizing creativity, imagination, and critical thinking to help individuals and organizations navigate uncertainty and complexity in an increasingly dynamic world(Department of the Prime Minister and Cabinet (DPMC), 2021). Given that Futures-thinking and design-thinking are complementary to one another, Roumiantseva, A. (2016), claims that they can be used in tandem to produce more comprehensive results.

Futures-thinking is important in design-thinking because it allows designers to anticipate and plan for potential changes, challenges, and opportunities that may arise in the future. Designers can produce more robust and sustainable solutions that satisfy users' needs in the long run by taking into account how a design solution will change and adapt over time.

Additionally, futures-thinking helps designers stay ahead of trends and innovations, ensuring that their designs remain relevant and competitive in a rapidly changing world. By envisioning possible future scenarios and outcomes, designers can make more informed decisions and design choices that align with their long-term goals and objectives.

- Characteristics of Futures-Thinking
- Steps involved in the Futures-Thinking Process

- Similarity of Design-Thinking and Futures-Thinking
- Design-Thinking vs Futures-Thinking

7.1 Characteristics of Futures-Thinking

Futures-thinking is a strategic and forward-looking approach that involves anticipating, preparing for, and adapting to future trends, uncertainties, and opportunities. Some key characteristics of Futures-thinking include:

7.1.1 Long-Term Perspective

Futures-thinking involves looking beyond short-term goals and immediate challenges to consider the long-term implications of current decisions and actions. It focuses on understanding how trends and developments today may shape the future. The long-term effects of greenhouse gas emissions, temperature increases, extreme weather, and sea level rise can be taken into account by decision makers when creating plans to cut carbon emissions, switch to renewable energy sources, strengthen the resilience of infrastructure, and adjust to shifting environmental conditions. To reduce emissions, improve green spaces, enhance public transportation, and get ready for more frequent and severe weather events, for example, a city government might create a long-term climate action plan with specific goals, targets, and actions. The city can create a more resilient and livable environment for its citizens now and in the future by being proactive and investing in sustainable policies and infrastructure.

7.1.2 Scenario Planning

Futures-thinking often involves creating and exploring different scenarios or future possibilities to prepare for a range of potential outcomes. By considering various scenarios, organizations can develop strategies that are flexible and adaptable to different futures. Examine a scenario planning exercise for a transportation company to see how they can anticipate and prepare for future market trends and changes. Based on various motivating factors, including consumer preferences, regulatory changes, technological advancements, and economic conditions, the company could develop several scenarios. Following are three fictitious situations:

- **Technological Disruption:** in this case, traditional car ownership is significantly reduced as a result of the quick developments in electric and driverless car technology. To provide on-demand autonomous vehicle services, the company will need to adapt by making investments in new technologies, forming alliances with tech firms, and rethinking its business strategy.

- **Climate Crisis:** in this scenario, traditional transportation infrastructure is disrupted by extreme weather events and rising sea levels brought on by climate change, which increases demand for sustainable transportation options. To lessen the effects of climate change, the business must concentrate on creating environmentally friendly transportation options, making investments in robust infrastructure, and working with governmental organizations.
- **Global Economic Recession:** in this scenario, consumer spending on transportation services declines as a result of a global economic recession. To attract clients during lean economic times, the business must simplify operations, reduce expenses, diversify its sources of income, and concentrate on offering value-added services.

The transportation company can discover possible risks and opportunities, decide on strategic investments and innovations, and forge resilience to face uncertain futures by creating and evaluating these scenarios. To survive in a quickly changing environment, scenario planning enables organizations to think strategically about the future, foresee obstacles, and proactively adjust to changing circumstances.

7.1.3 Strategic Foresight

Futures-thinking requires a strategic mindset that goes beyond predicting the future to actively shaping it. It involves identifying emerging trends, disruptions, and opportunities and developing strategies to capitalize on them. For a company specializing in machine learning and artificial intelligence (AI), a strategic foresight exercise would allow the business to anticipate future trends, identify new opportunities, and navigate potential challenges in the rapidly evolving AI landscape. These are some actions they could take:

- **Environmental Scanning:** the business would carry out a comprehensive examination of the external environment, covering the competitive landscape, market trends, technology developments, regulatory modifications, and societal transformations in artificial intelligence and machine learning. This would entail keeping an eye on industry reports, going to conferences, talking to professionals, and using data analytics tools to obtain information.
- **Trend Analysis:** the business would identify major trends influencing AI development going forward based on environmental scanning. These trends would include the emergence of explainable AI, ethical issues in AI research, the growing need for AI-powered solutions in the finance and healthcare sectors, and the effect of AI on job displacement. They would evaluate how these trends might affect their company and sector.

- **Scenario Development:** the business would create several scenarios showing various conceivable futures for the AI sector using the trends it had identified as building blocks. These scenarios could delve into a variety of possibilities, including the broad adoption of AI across all industries, regulatory pushback against AI, breakthrough discoveries in AI research, or unanticipated disruptions from new competitors.
- **Strategy Formulation:** the business would create strategic answers to every possible future based on the scenario analysis. This could entail making investments in R&D to remain at the forefront of AI innovation, forming alliances with other businesses to take advantage of complementary skills, creating a strong ethical framework for the application of AI, or broadening their product line to meet the demands of developing markets.

The technology company can position itself as a leader in a constantly evolving industry, foresee future opportunities and challenges in the AI landscape, and make well-informed decisions regarding resource allocation and strategic direction by adopting a strategic foresight for futures mindset. Organizations that possess strategic foresight are more comprehensive and able to stay resilient and competitive by actively shaping their future rather than just responding to external forces.

7.1.4 Systems Thinking

Futures-thinking takes a holistic approach by considering the interconnectedness of various factors and systems that influence the future. It involves understanding complex relationships and dynamics to anticipate potential impacts and consequences. Imagine a situation where a city is preparing for a future expansion and development while simultaneously tackling issues with resilience, sustainability, and quality of life.

- **Understanding the System:** the city begins by outlining the many interrelated systems—such as those related to housing, transportation, infrastructure, green spaces, social services, and the environment—that influence urban development. They take into account how these systems function within the urban ecosystem and affect one another.
- **Predicting Future Trends:** the city uses systems-thinking to predict future trends and scenarios, such as population growth, climate change, technological advancements, economic shifts, and social dynamics, that may have an impact on urban development. They analyze how these patterns might influence the course of the city in the future and point out possible obstacles and advantages.

- **Systems Mapping:** To illustrate the intricate connections and feedback loops among the various elements of the urban system, the city develops a systems map. They can more comprehensively grasp the system's interdependencies and leverage points by using this map, which can be used to target intervention or optimization efforts.
- **Scenario Planning:** the city uses scenario-planning to investigate various futures for urban development based on their comprehension of the system and future trends. They create several scenarios that take into consideration different risks and uncertainties, enabling them to test various plans of action under various circumstances.

By taking a comprehensive approach, they can improve both the environment and the well-being of their citizens while building cities that are ready to prosper in a world that is changing quickly.

7.1.5 Innovation and Creativity

Futures-thinking encourages creativity, innovation, and out-of-the-box thinking to envision new possibilities and solutions. It involves challenging assumptions, exploring unconventional ideas, and embracing experimentation. The creation of driverless vehicles is one instance of inventiveness. Self-driving cars, or autonomous vehicles, are a disruptive technology that could revolutionize urban mobility and the transportation sector in the future.

- **Visioning:** researchers and innovators have envisioned an autonomous vehicle-enabled transportation system that reduces traffic, increases road safety, and improves accessibility for people with mobility challenges. Through imagining a future in which autonomous vehicles coexist alongside conventional modes of transportation, stakeholders can develop a comprehensive vision for effective and sustainable urban mobility.
- **Technological Innovation:** the development of autonomous cars is being fueled by advances in data analytics, sensor technologies, artificial intelligence, and connectivity solutions. Stakeholders can hasten the development and implementation of safe, dependable, and efficient autonomous vehicles by funding research and development, encouraging interdisciplinary collaborations, and testing cutting-edge technologies in real-world settings.
- **Policy Innovation:** to guarantee public safety, data privacy, liability concerns, and ethical considerations are taken into account, policymakers are essential in forming the regulatory framework for autonomous vehicles. Governments can foster the adoption of autonomous vehicles and protect the interests of communities by formulating creative policies that strike a balance between innovation and societal concerns.

- **Business Model Innovation:** developing new revenue streams, alliances, and service offerings that take advantage of self-driving technology's capabilities is part of the process of innovating business models for autonomous vehicles. To meet the rising demand for autonomous driving solutions, businesses in the tech, mobility services, and automotive industries are experimenting with on-demand transportation services, shared mobility platforms, and subscription-based business models.
- **Social Innovation:** concerns about job displacement, accessibility, urban planning, and public acceptance are some of the significant social issues that autonomous vehicles bring up. To promote inclusivity, equity, and sustainability in the deployment of autonomous vehicles, stakeholders can encourage social innovation through community engagement, public consultations, and addressing concerns regarding the potential social effects of self-driving technology.
- **Cross-Sector Collaboration:** to propel innovation in autonomous vehicles, cooperation between automakers, tech firms, governmental organizations, academic institutions, and advocacy groups is crucial. Stakeholders can accelerate the global adoption of self-driving technology by overcoming technical obstacles, regulatory barriers, and market uncertainties through the sharing of knowledge, resources, and best practices across sectors.

To conclude, the advancement of self-driving cars serves as an example of how creativity and innovation in futures-thinking can result in revolutionary shifts in various sectors and communities. Stakeholders can influence a future in which autonomous vehicles contribute to a more sustainable, effective, and inclusive transportation ecosystem by adopting a forward-thinking mindset, utilizing cutting-edge technologies, encouraging collaboration across sectors, and addressing social implications.

7.1.6 Adaptability and Resilience

Futures-thinking recognizes the uncertainty and unpredictability of the future and emphasizes the importance of adaptability and resilience in the face of change. It involves being open to learning, adjusting strategies, and responding to unexpected developments. The reaction to the COVID-19 pandemic is one instance of Futures-thinking that demonstrates resilience and adaptability. People, organizations, and governments all over the world had to adjust swiftly to a rapidly shifting environment and an uncertain future when the pandemic struck in early 2020. During the pandemic, Futures-thinking demonstrated adaptability and resilience in the following ways:

- **Rapid Innovation:** scientists, researchers, and pharmaceutical companies worked together to quickly innovate and create new solutions in response to the pressing need for medical supplies, treatments, and vaccines. The rapidity with which vaccines were created and made available demonstrated the strength of flexibility and fortitude in responding to a major international emergency.
- **Remote Work and Digital Transformation:** many organizations had to swiftly adopt digital technologies and switch to remote work in order to continue operating when lockdowns and social distancing measures were put into place. Businesses that were able to modify their workflows and business models to fit into a virtual setting showed resilience in the face of change.
- **Scenario and Contingency Planning:** To anticipate potential pandemic outcomes and prepare for various contingencies, governments and healthcare systems participated in scenario planning exercises. Decision makers were able to lessen the impact of the crisis and adjust their plans in real-time by creating response plans based on various scenarios.
- **Community Resilience:** in the face of hardship, communities everywhere banded together to support one another during the pandemic. Individuals and groups worked together to provide vital services, resources, and emotional support to those in need through volunteer work and mutual aid networks.
- **Mental Health and Wellbeing Initiatives:** several organizations launched programs to enhance the mental health of their stakeholders and employees after realizing the pandemic's negative effects on mental health. Organizations showed resilience in providing care for their members during trying times by emphasizing mental health resources, encouraging work-life balance, and cultivating an environment of empathy and support.

All things considered, the COVID-19 pandemic response brought to light the significance of flexibility and resilience in forward-looking planning. Through the adoption of innovative and agile approaches, teamwork, scenario planning, and community assistance, people and institutions demonstrated resiliency and resolve in navigating an intricate and unpredictable future.

7.1.7 Collaboration and Diversity

Futures-thinking values diverse perspectives, expertise, and experiences to generate a more comprehensive understanding of future trends and possibilities. It involves fostering collaboration, dialogue, and co-creation to develop robust strategies that consider multiple viewpoints. The creation of inclusive and sustainable urban planning projects is one instance of cooperation and diversity in future thinking. There is a growing need for creative solutions that put environmental sustainability, social equity, and economic prosperity first as cities throughout the world struggle with issues related to rapid urbanization, climate change, and social inequality.

To co-create inclusive and resilient urban environments in this context, cooperation between a variety of stakeholders is crucial, including government agencies, urban planners, architects, community organizations, environmentalists, and residents. Together, these stakeholders possess a vast array of perspectives, expertise, and life experiences that they can draw from to create innovative and comprehensive urban planning strategies that tackle the multifaceted issues that cities face both now and in the future.

7.1.8 Continuous Learning

Futures-thinking involves a commitment to ongoing learning, reflection, and iteration. Organizations must stay informed about emerging trends, technologies, and market dynamics to proactively adapt their strategies. Scenario planning is one area where futures-thinking is demonstrating continuous learning. Using various realistic future scenarios based on various sets of assumptions and uncertainties, scenario planning is a strategic foresight technique. Organizations and decision makers can gain a better understanding of the opportunities and risks they may encounter and create more effective strategies to deal with uncertainty by investigating a variety of potential futures.

In scenario planning, continuous learning entails updating and improving scenarios regularly in response to fresh data, criticism, and insights. Organizations can stay flexible and resilient in the face of uncertainty by using this process to modify their strategies in response to evolving trends and changing conditions.

7.2 Steps Involved in Futures-thinking Processes

Futures-thinking involves a systematic approach to envisioning, planning, and preparing for potential future scenarios. Here are the steps involved in futures-thinking (Gandhi, S., 2017):

7.2.1 Choose a Specific Future

Selecting a specific future that is directly related to the process, organization, product, or service is the first step in the futures-thinking process. For example, the topic of discussion is to examine the particular future of "Smart Cities".

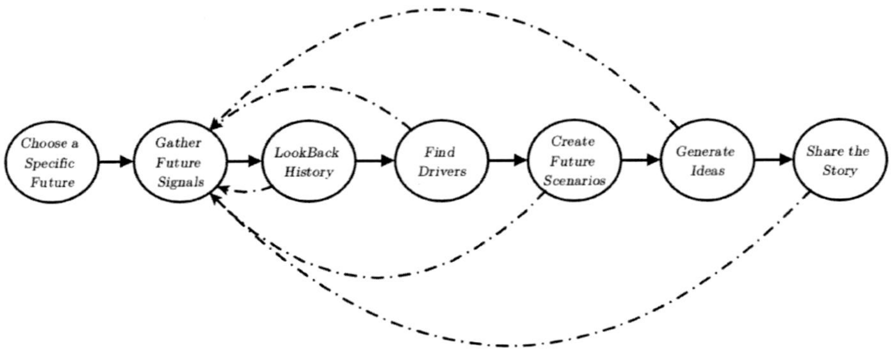

Figure 7.1: Futures-Thinking Steps

7.2.2 Gather Future Signals

Once the future is specified, identify the events (inventions, discoveries, policies, startups, etc) in the recent past that have a greater probability of affecting the chosen future. Look for signals of change related to smart cities, such as:

- **Advances in Technology:** keep an eye on developments in IoT (Internet of Things), AI (Artificial Intelligence), big data analytics, and blockchain that are driving smart city initiatives.
- **Urban Planning and Infrastructure:** monitor trends in sustainable architecture, transportation innovations, energy efficiency, and waste management practices in urban areas.
- **Government Policies and Regulations:** track changes in regulations related to data privacy, cybersecurity, and smart city governance that impact the development of smart cities.
- **Public Engagement and Citizen Participation:** Pay attention to initiatives promoting community involvement, digital inclusion, and social equity in smart city projects.

7.2.3 Look Back History

Identify the events in history that directly affected the field of the chosen future and signal. In the example, reflect on the historical context and evolution of smart cities to gain insights into past challenges, successes, and lessons learned:

- **Early Developments:** explore the origins of smart city concepts and initiatives, including pioneering projects that laid the foundation for urban innovation.
- **Case Studies:** examine successful smart city projects from around the world to understand the factors that contributed to their effectiveness and impact on urban development.

- **Challenges and Setbacks:** identify common obstacles faced by smart city initiatives, such as funding constraints, technological barriers, privacy concerns, and social disparities, and analyze how these challenges were addressed or mitigated over time.
- **Stakeholder Engagement:** review the roles of different stakeholders, including government agencies, private sector partners, academic institutions, and community organizations, in shaping the evolution of smart cities and fostering collaboration for sustainable urban development.

7.2.4 Find Drivers

Identify key drivers that are shaping the future of smart cities and urban development:

- **Technological Advancements:** explore emerging technologies such as artificial intelligence, Internet of Things (IoT), blockchain, and 5G networks that are transforming the way cities operate and deliver services to residents.
- **Environmental Sustainability:** consider the growing focus on sustainability, renewable energy, carbon footprint reduction, and climate change mitigation as key drivers influencing the development of smart cities.
- **Urbanization Trends:** analyze the impact of rapid urbanization, population growth, and migration on city infrastructure, transportation systems, housing affordability, and social equity, and how smart city solutions can address these challenges.
- **Data-driven Decision-Making:** examine the role of data analytics, big data, and predictive modeling in enabling cities to make informed decisions, optimize resource allocation, improve service delivery, and enhance citizen engagement.
- **Policy and Governance:** evaluate the importance of supportive policies, regulations, and governance structures in fostering innovation, collaboration, and partnerships among stakeholders to drive the successful implementation of smart city initiatives.

7.2.5 Create Future Scenarios

Based on the drivers and signals, simulate multiple possible scenarios that could happen in the future, which explores insights like advancements, changes, supports and constraints in the chosen field. By exploring these simulated scenarios based on the drivers and signals in smart cities and urban development, stakeholders can anticipate potential future outcomes, plan strategic interventions, and adapt to emerging trends to create more resilient, sustainable, and livable cities.

7.2.5.1 Scenario 1: Technological Innovation Drives Sustainable Urban Development

In this scenario, rapid advancements in technology, such as IoT, AI, and renewable energy solutions, lead to the widespread adoption of smart city initiatives focused on sustainability. Cities invest heavily in smart infrastructure, green buildings, electric transportation, and efficient waste management systems. Citizens benefit from cleaner air, reduced energy consumption, improved mobility options, and enhanced quality of life.

7.2.5.2 Scenario 2: Policy and Regulatory Changes Shape Smart City Development

Governments around the world introduce stringent regulations and policies to promote data privacy, cybersecurity, interoperability standards, and environmental protection in smart cities. This scenario leads to increased transparency, accountability, and trust among citizens and stakeholders. Cities prioritize citizen-centric services, open data initiatives, and ethical AI applications to build resilient and inclusive communities.

7.2.5.3 Scenario 3: Urbanization Challenges Drive Innovation in Smart City Solutions

Rapid urbanization and population growth pose significant challenges for cities in terms of infrastructure overload, traffic congestion, housing affordability, and social inequality. In response, cities leverage innovative technologies like autonomous vehicles, shared mobility services, vertical farming, and affordable housing solutions to address these urban challenges. Collaborative partnerships between government, industry, academia, and communities drive sustainable urban development.

7.2.5.4 Scenario 4: Citizen Engagement Transforms Urban Governance

Increasing citizen demands for participation, transparency, and inclusivity drive cities to adopt digital platforms, participatory budgeting mechanisms, and community-driven initiatives. Citizens become active co-creators of their urban environment, providing valuable insights, feedback, and ideas for improving services, infrastructure, and public spaces. This scenario fosters a sense of ownership, empowerment, and social cohesion among residents.

7.2.6 Generate Ideas

Use the scenarios that thinkers simulated to help come up with a fresh long-term strategy, vision, and future artifacts. To develop a fresh long-term strategy, vision, and future artifacts for smart cities and urban development, we can draw inspiration from the simulated scenarios created by thinkers. Here is a proposed approach:

7.2.6.1 Strategy

Based on the scenarios, the long-term strategy could benefit greatly from a focus on leveraging technological innovation, policy changes, urban challenges, and citizen engagement to drive sustainable urban development. The strategy could benefit greatly from prioritizing the following key areas:

- Sustainable infrastructure development
- Data privacy and cybersecurity measures
- Innovative solutions for urban challenges
- Citizen-centric governance and engagement

7.2.6.2 Vision

The vision for the future of smart cities should be centered around creating inclusive, resilient, and thriving urban communities. The vision statement could emphasize the following aspects:

- A connected and sustainable city ecosystem
- Empowered citizens shaping their urban environment
- A model for equitable and ethical urban development
- A hub for innovation and collaboration across sectors

7.2.6.3 Future Artifacts

To bring the vision to life, future artifacts can be conceptualized as tangible representations of the desired outcomes. These artifacts could include:

- Interactive smart city maps showcasing sustainable infrastructure projects
- Data privacy and cybersecurity guidelines for smart city governance
- Prototypes of innovative solutions for urban challenges (e.g., autonomous vehicles, vertical farming systems)
- Participatory budgeting platforms for citizen engagement in decision-making processes

By aligning the long-term strategy, vision, and future artifacts with the simulated scenarios, stakeholders can create a roadmap for implementing sustainable urban development initiatives that address current challenges and anticipate future trends. This holistic approach will help cities build resilient, inclusive, and innovative communities that prioritize the well-being of their residents.

7.2.7 Share the Story

Once at a correct strategy, vision, and future artifact, then share the story to introduce it to colleagues, clients, and customers.

7.3 Similarity of Design-Thinking and Futures-Thinking

Design-thinking and Futures-thinking share several similarities, as they both involve forward-looking and innovative approaches to problem-solving. Some key similarities between design-thinking and Futures-thinking include:

1. **Human-Centered Approach:** both design-thinking and futures-thinking prioritize understanding and addressing the needs and preferences of users or stakeholders. They emphasize empathy, research, and a deep understanding of human behavior to develop solutions that are relevant and meaningful.

2. **Creativity and Innovation:** design-thinking and futures-thinking encourage creative thinking and the exploration of new ideas to solve complex problems. They both involve divergent thinking to generate a wide range of possibilities and converge on innovative solutions.

3. **Iterative Process:** both approaches involve an iterative process of prototyping, testing, and refining ideas. design-thinking and futures-thinking recognize the importance of experimentation and learning from failures to continuously improve and innovate.

4. **Systems Thinking:** design-thinking and futures-thinking consider the broader context and interconnectedness of factors that influence a problem or opportunity. They both encourage a holistic approach to problem-solving that takes into account various perspectives and implications.

5. **Emphasis on Collaboration**: design-thinking and futures-thinking promote collaborative teamwork and interdisciplinary approaches to problem-solving. They recognize the value of diverse perspectives and expertise in generating creative solutions.

6. **Focus on Action and Implementation:** both approaches emphasize taking action and implementing solutions to create tangible impact. design-thinking and Futures-thinking seek to translate ideas into practical solutions that address real-world challenges.

The overall objective of design-thinking and futures-thinking is to support creativity, innovation, and forward-thinking methods of resolving complex issues and creating a more comprehensive future.

7.4 Design-Thinking vs Futures-Thinking

Although design-thinking and futures-thinking share some similarities in their approaches to problem-solving and innovation, they also have distinct differences in their focus and methodologies. Some key dissimilarities between design-thinking and Futures-thinking include.

Ultimately, the goal of Futures-thinking and design-thinking is to solve complex problems with creativity, innovation, and forward-thinking methods while creating a more comprehensive future.

7.5 Conclusion

Futures-thinking and design-thinking together provide a potent framework for taking on difficult problems and coming up with creative solutions. We can anticipate and plan for future changes and disruptions by incorporating Futures-thinking into the design process, which will make sure that our designs are flexible and long-lasting. Empathizing with users, defining issues, coming up with original solutions, prototyping and testing, and iterating in response to feedback are all encouraged by design-thinking. We are able to comprehend the possible effects of our designs in the context of changing trends, technologies, and societal changes when we integrate Futures-thinking into this process. By adopting this all-encompassing strategy, we can promote constructive change, mold a more sustainable future, and make a significant impact through intelligent and innovative design.

Table 7.1: Design-Thinking vs Futures-Thinking

	Design-Thinking	**Futures-Thinking**
Time Horizon	Design-thinking typically focuses on solving immediate and tangible problems, often related to improving existing products, services, or processes.	Futures-thinking is more concerned with anticipating and preparing for long-term trends, disruptions, and possibilities that may impact the future.
Scope of Impact	Design-thinking tends to have a narrower scope of impact, focusing on addressing specific user needs or challenges within a defined context.	Futures-thinking takes a broader perspective, considering macro-level trends, scenarios, and potential futures that may have far-reaching implications across industries and society.
Emphasis on Creativity vs. Strategic Foresight	Design-thinking places a strong emphasis on creativity, ideation, and prototyping to generate innovative solutions in a relatively short timeframe.	Futures-thinking, on the other hand, emphasizes strategic foresight, scenario planning, and trend analysis to anticipate and prepare for future uncertainties and opportunities.
Problem vs. Opportunity Orientation	Design-thinking is often problem-driven, seeking to identify and solve existing challenges or pain points for users.	Futures-thinking is more opportunity-oriented, exploring emerging trends, technologies, and possibilities to create new value and shape desired futures.
Stakeholder Engagement	Design-thinking focus on co-creating solutions with end-users and stakeholders in the present context.	Futures-thinking involves engaging a broader range of stakeholders to envision and shape future scenarios and strategies.
Methodologies and Tools	Design-thinking is typically associated with specific methodologies, such as the double diamond process or IDEO's design-thinking framework.	Futures-thinking may draw on various tools and techniques, such as scenario planning, trend analysis, horizon scanning, and backcasting to explore future possibilities and implications.

References

Department of the Prime Minister and Cabinet (DPMC). 2021. Futures thinking. https://www.dpmc.govt.nz/our-programmes/policy-project/policy-methods-toolbox/futures-thinking#:~:text=Futures%20thinking%20is%20a%20creative,right%20answer%20and%20reduce%20uncertainty. (Accessed: February 17, 2024).

Gandhi, S. 2017. Futures thinking and design thinking simply explained. https://bootcamp.uxdesign.cc/future-thinking-and-design-thinking-simply-explained-d65716d67651. (Accessed: February 20, 2024).

Roumiantseva, A. 2016. The fourth way: design thinking meets futures thinking. https://medium.com/@anna.roumiantseva/the-fourth-way-design-thinking-meets-futures-thinking-85793ae3aa1e. (Accessed: February 17, 2024).

Index

Made in the USA
Las Vegas, NV
15 September 2026

04eb322b-172e-498e-b00e-b6be32eeb0d8R02